Bioactive Proteins and Peptides from Marine Shellfish

Ming Du • Shuzhen Cheng
Editors

Bioactive Proteins and Peptides from Marine Shellfish

Springer

Editors
Ming Du
College of Food Science and Engineering
Dalian Ocean University
Dalian, China

Shuzhen Cheng
School of Food Science and Technology
Dalian Polytechnic University
Dalian, China

ISBN 978-981-95-3936-9 ISBN 978-981-95-3937-6 (eBook)
https://doi.org/10.1007/978-981-95-3937-6

This Springer imprint is published by the registered company Springer Nature Singapore Pte Ltd.
The registered company address is: 152 Beach Road, #21-01/04 Gateway East, Singapore 189721, Singapore

Foreword

In recent years, the development and utilization of marine biological resources has become a research hotspot in the fields of life and food science. In the vast treasure trove of the ocean, shellfish, with their rich species variation and large biomass, represent a rich source of high-quality proteins. The book *Bioactive Protein and Peptides from Marine Shellfish* focuses on the structure, chemistry, function, and application of marine shellfish proteins and peptides, systematically elucidating their basic research to their applied developments.

Professor Du Ming has been studying the field of marine biology for nearly two decades. With his groundbreaking academic achievements and extensive scientific research experience. Professor Du has in this book covered not only the key components about the structure, function, extraction, and separation technologies of marine shellfish proteins and peptides, but he has also explored the compositional characteristics of marine shellfish proteins, the activity mechanisms of their peptides, along with their flavor and processing characteristics. This book therefore provides both a solid theoretical foundation and practical guidance for related research as well as cutting-edge applications in multiple fields such as in food, medicine, and biological material applications.

This book represents a key reference for researchers engaged in the development of marine biological resources, for practitioners in the food and pharmaceutical industries, and for students interested in this field. It represents a comprehensive resource with an in-depth discussion on all aspects of marine shellfish proteins and peptides. It is envisaged that this book will propel new impetus into the research and industrial development of marine shellfish proteins and peptides while helping to harness the vast potential of marine biological resources, ultimately leading to novel advancements in both academic and practical applications.

Full Professor Emeritus, Department
of Biological Sciences, Faculty of Science & Engineering
University of Limerick,
Limerick, Ireland

R. J. FitzGerald

Foreword

Marine shellfish have a long history of use worldwide as a delicious and nutritious food, as well as a traditional medicine for various aliments among different cultures. As an important biological resource, marine shellfish are rich in protein, essential amino acids, healthy fatty acids, vitamins, and minerals, but low in saturated fat. In comparison to terrestrial proteins such as milk, egg, meat, and plant proteins, marine shellfish proteins show unique structures and functions. Over the past two decades, there is a growing interest in understanding the biological activities of marine shellfish proteins and their derived bioactive peptides. Therefore, a comprehensive reference book on marine shellfish bioactive proteins and peptides is more than timely.

The book titled *Bioactive Protein and Peptides from Marine Shellfish* is meticulously written by Professor Du Ming, an authoritative scholar in the field. Professor Du's research focuses on using cutting-edge technology to create healthy foods from shellfish. The book not only captures his latest research breakthroughs but also provides guidance for future research and innovation. The book first introduces recent advances in the molecular structure, physicochemical properties, and biological functions of marine shellfish proteins, and then discusses new developments on the methods of preparation, and structure-activity relationships of shellfish-derived bioactive peptides, and finally reveals recent trends in functional food development and application of bioactive ingredients.

This book covers both the theory and practice of chemistry, processing, bioactivity, and application of marine shellfish proteins and peptides, demonstrating a clear pathway for transforming laboratory fundamental discoveries into marketable products. This book will serve not only as a reference book for researchers, students, food developer, and educators but also as a scientific foundation to unlock the vast potential of marine shellfish. The publication is expected to stimulate new discovery and innovative uses of marine shellfish proteins and peptides in human health and other industries.

Jianping Wu

Professor, FIAFoST, FISNFF, FIFT, FAOCS,
FAGFD-ACS, Food Proteins and Bioactive
Peptides, Department of Agricultural,
Food and Nutritional Science
University of Alberta,
Edmonton, AB, Canada

Contents

About the Editors

Ming Du, PhD is a leading food scientist and President of Dalian Ocean University. He previously served as Vice President at Dalian Polytechnic University. He earned his PhD in Food Science from China Agricultural University and completed postdoctoral research at Harbin Institute of Technology.

His research focuses on protein bioactivity, functional peptides, and marine bioactive proteins. He has pioneered bioactive peptide identification and targeted hydrolysis technologies, contributing to functional food innovation. His work has resulted in over 200 SCI-indexed publications, including in *Nature Communications* and *ACS Nano*, 41 national invention patents, and multiple national science awards.

As the chief scientist of major national research projects, including a ¥40 million National Key R&D Project, he leads industry-academic collaborations in food science. He also directs the Liaoning Key Laboratory of Food Nutrition and Health and the Protein Science Division at Dalian Xinghai Bay Laboratory.

Beyond research, he serves as Editor-in-Chief of *eFood, Associate editor of Food Science and Human Wellness*, and on the editorial boards of several high-impact journals. He is also an expert advisor on national food industry committees, bridging scientific research and industrial applications in functional food development.

Shuzhen Cheng, PhD is an Associate Professor at Dalian Polytechnic University, specializing in marine bioactive peptides, functional foods, and precision nutrition. He earned his PhD in Food Science from China Agricultural University, where he was recognized as an Outstanding PhD Graduate of Beijing. Additionally, he completed a research fellowship at Leiden University Medical Center in the Netherlands, supported by the China Scholarship Council, focusing on the structure-function relationship of bioactive peptides.

His research explores the development and application of bioactive peptides for health promotion, with a focus on zinc absorption, anti-thrombosis, bone health, and fatigue resistance. His work has contributed to the high-value utilization of marine protein resources through an integrated screening, identification, and application approach. He has secured multiple national and provincial research grants, including funding from the National Natural Science Foundation of China and the National Key R&D Program.

He has published over 40 scientific papers in high-impact journals such as *Journal of Advanced Research, Journal of Agricultural and Food Chemistry*, *Critical Reviews in Food Science and Nutrition*, and *Trends in Analytical Chemistry*. He also holds several national patents related to bioactive peptide applications.

He serves on the youth editorial boards of *Agriculture Communications*, *Food and Health*, and *Journal of Future Food*. Actively engaged in industry collaboration, he leads functional food innovation projects with major food companies.

Abbreviations

1D-PAGE	One-dimensional polyacrylamide gel electrophoresis
2-DE	Two-dimensional electrophoresis
2D-PAGE	Two-dimensional polyacrylamide gel electrophoresis
5′-AMP	5′-Adenylic acid
5′-GMP	5′-Guanylic acid
5′-IMP	5′-Inosinic acid
AC	Affinity chromatography
ACE	Angiotensin-converting enzyme
ADA	Adenosine deaminase
ADP	Adenosine diphosphate
AK	Arginine kinase
AML12	Alpha mouse liver 12
AMP	Adenosine monophosphate
AMPs	Antimicrobial peptides
Ang I	Angiotensin I
Ang II	Angiotensin II
AP	Apical side
APCs	Antigen-presenting cells
APTT	Activated partial thromboplastin time
AT1	Angiotensin II type 1 receptor
AT-III	Antithrombin-III
ATP	Adenosine triphosphate
BL	Basolateral
BLI	Bio-layer interferometry
BMD	Bone mineral density
BMP	Beef meat peptide
BMP	Bone morphogenetic protein
BUN	Blood urea nitrogen
Ca^{2+}	Calcium ions
CALHM1	Calcium homeostasis modulator 1
CD	Circular dichroism spectroscopy

CDK	Cyclin-dependent kinase
CE	Electrophoresis methods
CE-QTOF-MS	Capillary electrophoresis tandem mass spectrometry
CHARMm	Chemistry at Harvard Macromolecular Mechanics
CID	Collision-induced dissociation
CLK	CDK-like kinase
CLSM	Confocal laser scanning microscopy
cTDA	Comparative taste dilution analysis
DBAASP	The Database of Antimicrobial Activity and Structure of Peptides
DH	Degree of hydrolysis
DHA	Docosahexaenoic acid
DSC	Differential scanning calorimetry
dsDNA	Double-stranded DNA
DXA	X-ray absorptiometry
EAST	Enzyme-allergy-susceptibility-absorption-test
ECE	Endothelin-converting enzyme
ELISA	Enzyme-linked immunosorbent assays
EPA	Eicosapentaenoic acid
ETD	Electron transfer dissociation
FCT	Fibrinogen clotting time
FICI	Fractional inhibitory concentration
FSH	Follicle-stimulating hormone
FT-IR	Fourier transform infrared spectroscopy
G Protein	Guanine nucleotide-binding protein
Glu	Glutamic acid
GnRH	Gonadotropin-releasing hormone
GPCRs	G protein-coupled receptors
GSK-3	Glycogen synthase kinase-3
HILIC	Hydrophilic interaction liquid chromatography
HK-2	Human proximaltubular epithelial cell line
HMM	Heavy meromyosin
HMWK	High molecular weight kininogen
HPH	High-pressure homogenization
HPLC	High-performance liquid chromatography
HPLC-MS	High-performance liquid chromatography mass spectrometry
HUVECs	Human umbilical vein endothelial cells
IEC	Ion exchange chromatography
IgE	Immunoglobulin E
IMAC	Immobilized metal affinity chromatography
L-AP4	L(+)-2-amino-4-phosphonobutanoic acid
LC	Liquid chromatography
LC-ESI-MS/MS	Liquid chromatography-tandem mass spectrometry
LC-MS	Liquid chromatography-mass spectrometry
LH	Luteinizing hormone

LMM	Light meromyosin
MALDI-QTOF-MS	Matrix-assisted laser desorption/ionization time-of-flight Mass spectrometer
MAPK	Mitogen-activated protein kinase
MFP	Myofibrillar proteins
Mfps	Mussel foot proteins
MHC	Myosin heavy chains
MHC-II	Major histocompatibility complex class II
MIM	Multiple ion monitoring
MLC	Myosin light chain
Mo-pt	Molybdopterin
MRM	Multiple reaction monitoring
MSG	monosodium glutamate
MSU	Monosodium urate
Na^+	Sodium ions
NAY	N-(9,10-anthraquinone-2-ylcarbonyl) xanthine oxidase inhibitors
NO	Nitric oxide
NSAIDs	Nonsteroidal anti-inflammatory drugs
O	Oxygen
OAS	Oral allergy syndrome
OPG	Osteoclastogenesis inhibitory factor
PAGE	Polyacrylamide gel electrophoresis
PAI-1	Plasminogen activator inhibitor-1
PCA	Polymerase chain reaction
PDE	Phosphodiesterases
PGI2	Prostacyclin
pI	Isoelectric point
PK	Prekallikrein
PMF	Peptide mass fingerprinting
pNA	P-nitroaniline
PO	Potassium oxonate
PT	Prothrombin time
PVDF	Polyvinylidene fluoride
Q-IT	Quadrupole ion trap
QSAR	Quantitative structure-activity relationship
Q-TOF	Quadrupole time-of-flight
RANK	Receptor activator for nuclear factor-κB
RANKL	Receptor activator for nuclear factor-κB ligand
RAS	Renin-angiotensin system
ROS	Reactive oxygen species
RP-HPLC	Reversed-phase high-performance liquid chromatography
RP-UHPLC	Reversed-phase ultra-high-performance liquid chromatography
RUNX2	Runt-related transcription factor 2
S	Sulfur

S1	Subfragment 1
SAR	Structure-activity relationship
SCP	Sarcoplasmic protein
SCr	Serum creatinine
SDI	Socio-demographic indices
SDS-PAGE	Polyacrylamide gel electrophoresis
SDS-PAGE	Sodium dodecyl sulfate-polyacrylamide gel Electrophoresis
SEC	Size exclusion chromatography
Ser	Serine
SHR	Spontaneously hypertensive rats
SIM	Selected ion monitoring
SPR	Surface plasma resonance
SPT	Skin prick test
SUA	Serum uric acid
T1R1/T1R3	Taste receptor type 1 member 1 and Taste receptor type 1 member 3
TAV	Taste activity value
TD	Taste dilution
TDA	Taste dilution analysis
TEM	Transmission electron microscopy
TGase	Transglutaminase
TM	Thrombomodulin
TNBS	Trinitrobenzenesulfonic acid
TNF-α	Tumor necrosis factor-alpha
TRACP5b	Tartrate-resistant acid phosphatase 5b
TRCs	Transient receptor potential canonical channels
TRPM5	Transient receptor potential channel M5
UF	Ultrafiltration
UHPH	Ultra-high pressure homogenization
UPLC-QTOF-MS	Ultra-performance liquid chromatography time-of-flight Mass spectrometry
UV	Ultraviolet
VFTD	Venus flytrap domain
VSM	Vibrating sample magnetometer
vWF	Von Willebrand factor
XO	Xanthine oxidase
XOI	Xanthine oxidase inhibitors
XRD	X-ray powder diffraction

Chapter 1
Introduction

Ming Du, Shuzhen Cheng, Hui Chen, and Xinran Liu

Abstract The ocean covers 71% of the Earth's surface and hosts a vast reservoir of biological resources. Shellfish, particularly marine bivalves and gastropods, represent a significant component of these resources, holding high nutritional and economic value. Global fisheries and aquaculture production reached a record 223.2 million tons in 2022, with shellfish aquaculture playing a major role. China is the world's largest producer, contributing 70% of global shellfish output. Shellfish are rich in proteins, peptides, unsaturated fats, minerals, and vitamins, and possess various bioactive properties, such as antihypertensive, antithrombotic, and bone-health-promoting effects. Furthermore, enzymatic hydrolysis of shellfish proteins can yield bioactive peptides with broad application potential. Despite challenges in aquaculture, including stringent seedling requirements and water safety standards, technological advances and selective breeding offer promising pathways for sustainable development.

Keywords Marine Shellfish · Global Resources · Aquaculture · Nutritional Value · Bioactive Peptides

M. Du (✉)
College of Food Science and Engineering, Dalian Ocean University, Dalian, China

S. Cheng
School of Food Science and Technology, Dalian Polytechnic University, Dalian, China

H. Chen
Food Science and Engineering, Zhejiang University of Technology, Zhejiang, China

X. Liu
Food Science and Engineering, Dalian Polytechnic University, Dalian, China

M. Du, S. Cheng (eds.), *Bioactive Proteins and Peptides from Marine Shellfish*,
https://doi.org/10.1007/978-981-95-3937-6_1

1.1 Global Marine Shellfish Resources

The State of World Fisheries and Aquaculture (SOFIA) report, released by the Food and Agriculture Organization of the United Nations (FAO) in 2024, revealed that global fisheries and aquaculture production reached 223.2 million tons. Of this total, 185.4 million tons were aquatic animals, and 37.8 million tons were algae. In 2021, global apparent consumption of aquatic animal food stood at 162.5 million tons, nearly twice the rate of global population growth since 1961. Meanwhile, global per capita annual consumption of aquatic animals rose from 9.1 kg in 1961 to 20.7 kg in 2022. Within the total aquatic animal output, 89% is used for direct human consumption, underscoring the critical role of fisheries and aquaculture in safeguarding global food security. The remaining 11% is allocated to indirect or nonfood uses, primarily for producing fish meal and fish oil. Geographically, Asian countries accounted for 70% of global aquatic animal production from fisheries and aquaculture in 2022, followed by Europe, Latin America and the Caribbean, Africa, North America, and Oceania. China remains the world's largest fishery producer, trailed by India, Indonesia, Vietnam, and Peru. Over the past 2 years, the aquaculture sector has grown at a faster pace than the capture fisheries sector.

Global production and apparent consumption of aquatic products are projected to rise by 2032. Specifically, aquatic animal output is expected to increase by 10% to reach 205 million tons by that year, driven primarily by the expansion of aquaculture scales and the recovery of capture fisheries production. However, recent fishing output has declined to 90.3 million tons, representing a 4.0% decrease compared to the average level of the previous three years. As shown in Table 1.1, in the global marine mollusk catch in 2020, the output of scallop in bivalves was 357,000 tons, accounting for 6% of the total amount of mollusks, and the total output of other mollusks was 24.78 million tons. In 2020, the global marine mollusk aquaculture output was 17.74 million tons, of which oysters ranked first with 545,000 tons, accounting for 31% of the total mollusk aquaculture output, clams and scallops were 4.27 million tons and 1.75 million tons, respectively, accounting for the second and third place of the total output (Table 1.2).

According to FAO statistics in 2020, China's output of marine bivalves was 47.5591 million tons, far exceeding that of other countries or regions in the world, such as Chile (1.2661 million tons), Japan (642,900 tons), South Korea (568,400 tons), and the United States (468,200 tons) (Table 1.3) [1].

China stands as the world's largest shellfish farming nation, contributing 70% of global total shellfish production. According to the 2023 China Fishery Statistical Yearbook, China's total shellfish output in 2022, encompassing both marine and freshwater shellfish products, reached 15.6958 million tons, accounting for 33.8% of the country's total aquaculture production. This underscores the pivotal role of shellfish in China's fishery economy. There are more than 800 species of marine shellfish in China, including more than 60 species of major economic shellfish, including *Crassostrea gigas*, *Haliotis gigantean*, *Patinopecten yessoensi*s, and *Mytilu edulis* [2].

Table 1.1 Global marine mollusk catch

Species	Production (kt)							Various proportions in 2020 (%)
	2004–2013	2015	2016	2017	2018	2019	2020	
Dosidicus gigas	823	1004	747	763	892	914	877	15
Mollusca	802	759	674	644	658	707	600	10
Loliginidae and *Ommastrephidae*	641	693	629	655	571	614	529	9
Sepiidae and *Sepiolidae*	301	405	379	395	347	365	353	6
Cephalopoda	382	388	394	433	322	425	424	7
Mizuhopecten yessoensis	309	243	224	247	316	351	357	6
Else	3110	3279	2361	2486	2549	2624	2438	41
Total	6616	7129	5728	5960	5956	6171	5923	100

*Data sources: The State of World Fisheries and Aquaculture 2022

Table 1.2 Global marine mollusk aquaculture output

Species	Production (kt)						Various proportions in 2020(%)
	2010	2012	2014	2016	2018	2020	
Crassostrea spp.	3570	3807	4181	4690	5171	5450	31
Ruditapes philippinarum	3500	3618	3838	4175	4139	4266	24
Pectinidae	1366	1360	1576	1849	1918	1746	10
Mytilidae	871	937	992	1085	1205	1108	6
Sinonovacula constricta	693	690	752	799	852	860	5
Magallana gigas	640	609	623	573	643	610	3
Anadara granosa	456	378	434	430	433	458	3
Mytilus chilensis	221	244	238	300	365	400	2
Total	13,728	14,346	1570	16,840	17,510	17,742	100

*Data sources: The State of World Fisheries and Aquaculture 2022

Table 1.3 Main cultivation and production countries of bivalves

Major breeding producing countries	Total output(kt)	Bivalve production(kt)	Proportion(%)
China	47559.1	13358.3	28.1
Chile	1266.1	376.9	29.8
Japan	642.9	350.4	54.5
Republic of Korea	568.4	391.1	68.8
The United States	468.2	181.1	38.7
Spain	347.8	287	82.5
Taiwan Province of China	283.2	75.8	26.8
Canada	191.3	43.2	22.6
France	185.2	144.8	78.2
Italy	143.3	93.2	65
New Zealand	104.5	88.2	84.3

*Data sources: The State of World Fisheries and Aquaculture 2020

1.2 Economic Value and Prospects of Marine Shellfish

According to the 2024 State of World Fisheries and Aquaculture report, global fisheries and aquaculture production reached a historic high in 2022, totaling 223.2 million tons, with aquatic animals accounting for 185.4 million tons of this figure. Breaking down the total output by source, 62% originated from marine environments, where 69% came from capture fisheries and 31% from aquaculture. The remaining 38% came from inland waters, with 84% derived from aquaculture and 16% from capture fisheries. However, there are huge differences in production among regions, subregions, and countries. Aquatic animal production in Asian countries accounted for 70% of the total production, followed by Europe, Latin America and the Caribbean (all 9%), Africa (7%), North America (3%), and Oceania (1%). In 2022, China continued to maintain its position as a major producer, accounting for 36% of the total output, followed by India (8%), Indonesia (7%), Vietnam (5%), and Peru (3%).

1.2.1 Economic Value

From 1976 to 2020, the nominal annual growth rate of global aquatic product trade value averaged 6.9%, with an actual growth rate of 3.9%. Among shellfish, scallops, clams, oysters, and mussels are the primary commodities in international trade. In 2020, global exports of bivalve mollusks totaled US $4.3 billion, accounting for approximately 2.8% of the world's total aquatic product export value. The FAO predicts that over the next decade, production, consumption, and trade in fisheries and aquaculture will continue to increase, albeit at a slower growth rate. Driven by the sustained expansion of aquaculture, global aquaculture output is projected to reach 100 million tons for the first time in 2027 and 106 million tons by 2030. Meanwhile, total aquatic animal production is expected to hit 202 million tons by 2030. Currently, the vast majority of consumed bivalve mollusks are farmed, with key producing countries and regions, including Europe, North America, China, and Chile. Import demand is dominated by the European Union, the United States, China, and South Korea. In recent years, international market demand for bivalves has remained relatively stable, and they have gradually emerged as a healthy and sustainable food choice.

1.2.2 Development

Bivalve mollusks provide balanced, bioaccessible nutrients to support healthy and active lifestyles, while aquaculture activities enhance the livelihoods of coastal communities. Thus, bivalve aquaculture plays a vital role in "nutrition-sensitive" aquatic food systems, social systems that deliver diverse, nutritionally comprehensive foods and foster sustainable livelihoods. In addition, growing recognition has emerged around the broader ecosystem benefits of coastal bivalve aquaculture, including carbon sequestration, nutrient cycling, coastal protection, and other ecosystem services. Since bivalve aquaculture does not require external feeding, it has minimal reliance on artificial feed and lower operational costs. Despite the general accessibility and affordability of bivalve aquaculture technologies, however, global development in this sector remains relatively slow. Key constraints include two primary factors. Firstly, stringent requirements for bivalve seedlings, particularly for the export market. Second, rigorous testing and product safety standards for harvesting waters in bivalve aquaculture. Over the past two decades, global bivalve production has merely doubled. Pacific oysters and Philippine clams dominate bivalve output, followed by scallops and mussels. Meanwhile, additional challenges such as climate change, the COVID-19 pandemic, shellfish diseases, extreme weather events, and long-term financial constraints all hamper the development of shellfish and other aquatic organisms.

1.2.3 Prospect

Given the stringent requirements for bivalve seedlings in aquaculture, nursery design and technology have advanced significantly in recent years, particularly in domestication, spawning, larval rearing, and seeding, with concurrent improvements in larval survival rates. Computer-aided monitoring and optimization of larval feed have further enhanced phytoplankton production in nurseries, which in turn has boosted larval survival and growth rates. Advances in refined seeding processes and materials allow farmers to produce seedlings tailored to specific needs, while improved material handling has facilitated large-scale seeding and colonization, particularly for oysters. In addition, shellfish aquaculture has benefited from selective breeding efforts and the development of strains and varieties with enhanced disease resistance and rapid growth. Continued research and technological innovation in bivalve aquaculture have opened new frontiers to support the global expansion of sustainable aquaculture.

1.3 Marine Shellfish

Shellfish meat is not only delicious but also highly nutritious, making it popular among consumers of all ages. Research has shown that shellfish are rich in various bioactive components, including taurine, proteins, and peptides, which endow them with significant health benefits and medicinal value. In China, aquaculture production or experimental cultivation is currently underway for over 60 major economic shellfish species. Among these, more than 20 species, such as oysters, mussels, clams, scallops, and abalone, have already achieved large-scale farming.

1.3.1 Nutritional Composition

1.3.1.1 Water

Water is an essential nutrient in any living system. On average, adults have about 60% water in their bodies. Even if dehydration accounts for only 2% of body weight, it will cause adverse physiological reactions. Water is the biochemical solvent of the body and is necessary to maintain body temperature. Fresh marine shellfish contain about 75% water.

1.3.1.2 Protein

Protein is the most important nutrient for the human body. Proteins are composed of essential and nonessential amino acids. Amino acids are also precursors for the synthesis of nucleic acids, enzymes, hormones, and other substances. Marine shellfish are rich in protein, which is comparable to land-based protein sources. For example, the protein content in clams, mussels, oysters, and scallops is 9.0–13.0%, 12.6–13.0%, 8.9–14.3%, and 14.8–17.7%, respectively. The essential amino pattern of marine shellfish is considered a high-quality protein source because of its high digestibility.

1.3.1.3 Carbohydrate

Carbohydrates in food, such as sugar, fiber, and starch, are converted into glucose, which quickly provides energy for the body. In general, terrestrial and aquatic protein sources exist almost in the form of glycogen. The tissues of mollusks and shellfish contain moderate levels of carbohydrates, and the tissues of scallops, oysters, and mussels contain 3–5% carbohydrates.

1.3.1.4 Fat

Fat is the main source of energy stored in the human body. Edible fats and oils exist in the form of triglycerides in the natural state and are composed of three fatty acids connected to the glycerol backbone. Compared with land-based meat (3.6–18.7 g/100 g), mollusk shellfish have a low fat content (0.96–4.5 g/100 g). Compared with chicken, pork, or beef (1–7.3 g/100 g), its saturated fat content is also significantly lower (1 g/100 g). Omega-3 fatty acids, including α-linolenic acid, eicosapentaenoic acid (EPA), and docosahexaenoic acid (DHA), are considered to play a major role in human health. Nutritional suggestions on the intake of omega-3 fatty acids mainly focus on oily fish, but mussels and oysters are also good sources of omega-3 total fatty acids. Different species have different types of fatty acids, and shellfish are rich in EPA and DHA. The total amount of omega-3 fatty acids in oysters is more than 500 mg/100 g, but scallops almost do not contain omega-3 fatty acids.

1.3.1.5 Cholesterol

In general, the cholesterol content of marine shellfish is lower than that of beef, chicken, or pork. Researchers also reported that oysters and other mollusks have relatively low cholesterol levels. The cholesterol content of Oriental oyster (30 mg/100 g) was slightly lower than that of Pacific oyster (48 mg/100 g). The cholesterol content of steamed oysters was the highest, followed by fresh and canned oysters, which were 56 mg/100 g, 28 mg/100 g, and 3 mg/100 g, respectively.

1.3.1.6 Mineral

The calcium content in shellfish is 2–10 times higher than that in beef, chicken, or pork. Oysters (4.6–5.8 mg/100 g) and mussels (95 mg/100 g) are excellent sources of iron. Clam (1.62 mg/100 g) has less iron than oyster, but it is still a good source of iron. Fried scallops are also a good source of magnesium, containing about 18–58 mg/100 g, while other mollusk shellfish contain 14–37 mg/100 g [3].

1.3.1.7 Vitamin

The vitamin C content of marine shellfish is more prominent, and the vitamin C content of oyster tissue can reach 8 mg/100 g. In addition, there is high taurine in oysters, and the taurine of different kinds of oysters reaches 1.0–1.2 g/100 g. The content of other vitamins in shellfish is generally [4].

1.3.2 Shellfish Organization

The tissue structure of shellfish primarily comprises the mantle, gills, digestive glands, liver, reproductive glands, ventricle, and adductor muscle, among other organs. The mantle, located in the outermost layer, secretes the hard shell that protects the shellfish from external damage. Inside the mantle lie the gills, which serve dual functions of respiration and food filtration. Shellfish possess well-developed gills capable of filtering large volumes of seawater to extract nutrients. The digestive glands are responsible for digesting and absorbing nutrients, while the intestine further breaks down and absorbs food to supply additional energy and essential substances. The liver acts as a key organ for digestion and metabolism in shellfish, breaking down, absorbing, and converting nutrients from food into the energy and materials required for bodily functions. Reproductive glands are sexually dimorphic. Female reproductive glands produce eggs, whereas male ones generate sperm. The ventricle functions as a blood-pumping organ, transporting blood throughout the body to sustain the normal operation of various tissues and organs. The adductor muscle, a contractile muscle located at both ends of the shell, controls the opening and closing of the shell. When threatened or in need of protection, shellfish contract their adductor muscles to seal the shell tightly, thereby avoiding external harm.

1.3.3 Bioactive Peptides

Marine shellfish are rich in protein and play a pivotal role in aquatic protein production. Boasting broad market value and development potential, they have become a key research focus for the future. However, natural shellfish contain high levels of endogenous autolytic enzymes, resulting in a short shelf life. Thus, research into shellfish protein processing holds significant practical importance [5]. Currently, marine shellfish are primarily hydrolyzed into peptides using proteases to enhance their high-value utilization. Bioactive peptides are protein degradation fragments, typically consisting of amino acid sequences ranging from 2 to 20 residues in length. These peptides can be obtained through enzymatic hydrolysis or released during gastrointestinal digestion and/or food processing. Beyond serving as sources of nitrogen and amino acids, peptides exert various physiological functions in the body. Specifically, peptides derived from marine shellfish have been reported to possess multiple biological activities, including antihypertensive, antithrombotic, bone-promoting effects, and taste-enhancing properties.

Currently, research on the development of bioactive peptides from marine shellfish protein resources in China primarily focuses on utilizing major shellfish species such as oysters, scallops, and clams [4]. The production and preparation of bioactive peptides from shellfish mainly involve two approaches. First, directly extracting naturally occurring bioactive peptides from shellfish tissues. Second, degrading marine shellfish proteins using biological enzymes to obtain peptides with specific physiological activities. To date, nearly several thousand types of bioactive peptides have been reported. This book will systematically elaborate on the preparation, identification, and biological activity studies of shellfish-derived peptides. In recent years, both domestic and international research on active peptides from shellfish has been increasing. However, progress in their practical development remains limited. Therefore, this book summarizes the latest research status of marine shellfish proteins and bioactive peptides at home and abroad in recent years, aiming to provide references for their high-value transformation.

References

1. Zhu BW. Research on processing theory and technology of seafood treasures. Beijing: Science Press; 2010. (in Chinese).
2. Peng D, Zhang S, Zhang H, Pang D, Yang Q, Jiang R, Lin Y, Mu Y, Zhu Y. The oyster fishery in China: trend, concerns and solutions. Mar Policy. 2021;129:104524.
3. Hummel M, Talsma EF, Taleon V, Londoño L, Brychkova G, Gallego S, Raatz B, Spillane C. Iron, zinc and phytic acid retention of biofortified, low phytic acid, and conventional bean varieties when preparing common household recipes. Nutrients. 2020;12(3):658.
4. Wright AC, Fan Y, Baker GL. Nutritional value and food safety of bivalve molluscan shellfish. J Shellfish Res. 2018;37(4):695–708.
5. Qi-men Z. Research progress in shellfish preservation technology, 2014.

Chapter 2
Molecular Composition and Characteristics of Marine Shellfish Protein

Ming Du, Shuzhen Cheng, Hongrui Chen, and Weiwei Fan

Abstract With the increasing demand for protein worldwide, marine shellfish protein has attracted more and more attention because of its large yield and high nutritional value. To date, the output of shellfish aquaculture in China has continued to grow. The sustainable development of marine shellfish protein has become a hot topic. To improve the deep-processing level of marine shellfish proteins, the molecular composition and characteristics of marine shellfish proteins were reviewed in this chapter. In particular, the marine shellfish protein composition, amino acid composition, temperature stability, pH stability, and ion-binding properties are involved. These are expected to provide new ideas for the practical application of marine shellfish proteins in the medical and food industries.

Keywords Marine shellfish protein · Amino acid · Temperature stability · pH stability · Ion-binding properties

Shellfish, belonging to the phylum Mollusca, are a group of marine organisms of great concern. In recent years, with the continuous development of artificial breeding technology, the output of shellfish aquaculture in China has continued to increase, and the production of marine bivalve shellfish in China in 2020 was 47.5591 million tons [1]. There are many kinds of farmed shellfish in China, including *Chlamys farreri*, *Bay scallops*, *Mizuhopecten yessoensis*, *Mytilus edulis*, *Mytilus unguiculatus*, *Crassostrea gigas*, *Ruditapes philippinarum*, *Tegillarca granosa*, *Sinonovacula constricta*, and *Haliotis discus hannai ino*. Shellfish protein is an

M. Du (✉)
College of Food Science and Engineering, Dalian Ocean University, Dalian, China

S. Cheng
School of Food Science and Technology, Dalian Polytechnic University, Dalian, China

H. Chen
Food and Bioengineering, XiHua University, Chengdu, China

W. Fan
Biological Engineering, Dalian Polytechnic University, Dalian, China
e-mail: fanww@dlpu.edu.cn

M. Du, S. Cheng (eds.), *Bioactive Proteins and Peptides from Marine Shellfish*,
https://doi.org/10.1007/978-981-95-3937-6_2

important source of seafood protein and has high nutritional value because of its rich variety, large resources, and complete amino acids.

2.1 Marine Shellfish Protein Composition

2.1.1 Overview of Marine Shellfish Protein

Shellfish muscle proteins can be categorized into water-soluble proteins, salt-soluble proteins, and insoluble proteins based on their differences in solubility [2]. Water-soluble proteins, also referred to as sarcoplasmic proteins, are a collective term for various proteins soluble in water (or dilute salt solutions) within the sarcoplasm of muscle cells. These proteins contain numerous metabolism-related zymoproteins and primarily influence the taste and color characteristics of shellfish meat. Salt-soluble proteins (myofibrillar proteins) are complexes composed of myosin, actin, actomyosin, and regulatory proteins. They are closely linked to the water-holding capacity, emulsifying properties, and gelling ability of meat. Insoluble proteins (muscle matrix proteins), including collagen and elastin, are the residual fraction after removing water-soluble and salt-soluble proteins. As key components of connective tissue, they are associated with the tenderness and elasticity of shellfish meat [3]. While the content of these three protein types varies slightly across different shellfish species, myofibrillar proteins dominate the muscle composition in most shellfish.

Myofibrillar protein is a key structural protein in animals, primarily responsible for muscle contraction. It is mainly composed of thin filaments and thick filaments, and muscle contraction is achieved through the mutual sliding of these two types of filaments [2]. In shellfish muscle protein, thin filaments are built around actin. Tropomyosin and troponin are located in the spiral grooves of the actin helix, together forming the thin filament structure. Shellfish thick filaments, also called "crude myosin" or paramyosin filaments, consist mainly of paramyosin, myosin, and twitchin. Paramyosin molecules aggregate to form a rod-like core, with myosin regularly attached to the outer surface of this core. The myosin head contains ATPase activity, which provides energy for filament sliding by breaking down ATP (Fig. 2.1) [4].

In addition to striated muscle, shellfish muscle contains smooth muscle and paramyosin. Paramyosin is a unique myofibrillar protein in invertebrates, closely related to the specialized movements of bivalve adductor muscles. It is particularly abundant in bivalve adductor muscles, accounting for over 50% of myofibrillar proteins in the scallop adductor muscle. In shellfish smooth muscle, the structure of thin and thick filaments is very similar to that of striated muscle. However, myorod protein is present in smooth muscle but absent in striated muscle, making it a marker protein to distinguish between the two muscle types [5]. Paramyosin constitutes more

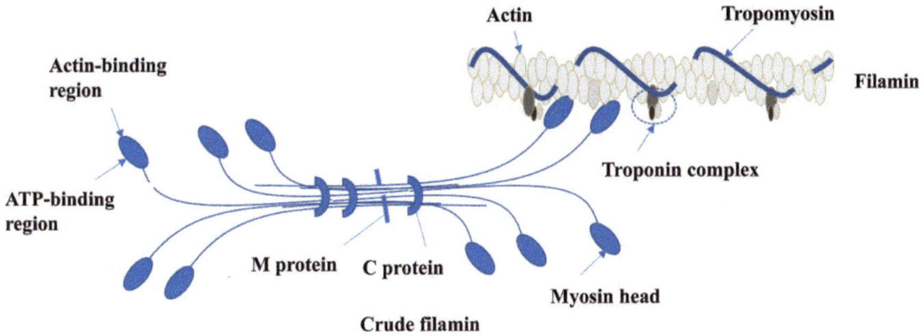

Fig. 2.1 Structure diagram of myofibrillar protein

than 80% of the thick filament proteins in smooth muscle and is located at its core, thus earning smooth muscle the name "paramyosin smooth muscle." In contrast, in the striated muscle myofibrillar proteins of *Chlamys nipponensis*, myosin content exceeds 50%, while paramyosin accounts for only about 5%. In smooth muscle, both myosin and paramyosin each make up approximately 30% of myofibrillar proteins. Similarly, the paramyosin content in the smooth muscle of *Zygochlamys patagonica* is significantly higher than in its striated muscle [6].

2.1.2 Oyster

Oysters rank among China's four major cultured shellfish. They are not only rich in nutrients, including protein (39.1–53.1%), taurine, glycogen, vitamins, and trace elements like copper, iron, and zinc, but also serve as an excellent source of food protein. In terms of protein solubility, water-soluble proteins have the highest content at 37.79%, followed by salt-soluble proteins (31.10%) and insoluble proteins (26.44%). The molecular weight distribution of oyster proteins treated with β-mercaptoethanol differs significantly from that of untreated samples, treated samples exhibit more protein bands in electrophoresis. Specifically, water-soluble proteins in treated samples show continuous distribution across the 200–14 kDa range, while salt-soluble proteins are mainly concentrated between 200 and 10 kDa. Key components in this range include myosin heavy chain (200 kDa), actin (45 kDa), and paramyosin typically around 97 kDa. Insoluble proteins in treated samples distribute across 200–29 kDa. In contrast, the electrophoretic profile of untreated oyster proteins shows distinct patterns. Water-soluble proteins mainly concentrate at 116 kDa, salt-soluble proteins primarily distribute at 200 kDa and 116 kDa, and insoluble proteins appear at 36 kDa and 29 kDa [7].

2.1.3 Scallop

Scallops are nutrient-rich seafood, packed with protein, phosphorus, calcium, iron, iodine, and various vitamins. Their primary edible part is the adductor muscle, where the protein content in fresh scallop adductor muscle reaches approximately 19%, with actomyosin as the main functional protein. Scallop muscle consists of two types, which are striated muscle (mainly distributed in the adductor muscle) and smooth muscle (primarily in the mantle). Scallop muscle proteins are categorized into sarcoplasmic proteins, myofibrillar proteins, and myostromal proteins, among which myofibrillar proteins account for the largest proportion. Notably, levels of myosin heavy chain and paramyosin differ slightly between the two muscle types. Myosin heavy chain makes up 30.5% of striated muscle but only 17.6% of smooth muscle, while paramyosin content is lower in striated muscle (11.53%) than in smooth muscle (31.15%). Combined, myosin and paramyosin account for about 50% of the protein in both muscle types. The ratio of paramyosin to myosin heavy chain is 0.38 in striated muscle compared to 1.77 in smooth muscle. In terms of myosin content alone, striated muscle contains 9.91%, slightly higher than smooth muscle's 8.83%. Additionally, smooth muscle contains 5.04% myorod, a protein specific to smooth muscle tissue [8].

Sodium dodecyl sulfate-polyacrylamide gel electrophoresis (SDS-PAGE) was used to analyze myofibrillar proteins and sarcoplasmic proteins in the adductor muscles and mantles of three scallop species, *Mizuhopecten yessoensis*, bay scallops (*Argopecten irradians*), and *Chlamys farreri*. Sarcoplasmic proteins exhibited more bands than myofibrillar proteins across all samples. Within the same scallop species, adductor muscles contained more protein bands than mantles. Key protein bands, corresponding to myosin heavy chain, actin, tropomyosin, and paramyosin, were primarily distributed around 200 kDa, 42 kDa, 35 kDa, and 100 kDa, respectively, across the three scallop species. Sarcoplasmic proteins showed numerous bands, mainly concentrated in the 90–160 kDa and 35–55 kDa ranges. In addition, scallop mantles are rich in protein, including a certain amount of collagen. Type I fibrous collagen is the most abundant and widely studied collagen type. In vertebrates such as fish, it typically consists of two $\alpha1$ (I) chains and one $\alpha2$ (I) chain. For the three scallop species, collagen bands in the outer membrane were mainly distributed in the 212–185 kDa range, corresponding to β-peptide chains. However, α-peptide chain bands in the 158–116 kDa range were not distinct in the three scallop species [9].

2.1.4 Mussel

Mussels are both delicious and nutritious, earning them the nickname "eggs of the sea" due to their high protein content. The protein content of dried mussels reaches approximately 55–60% [10]. Among mussel proteins, water-soluble proteins are the most abundant, followed by salt-soluble proteins and acid-soluble matrix proteins. Water-soluble protein bands in mussels are primarily distributed at 16.76, 26.68, 29.51, 35.53, and 38.11 kDa. Salt-soluble proteins show prominent bands at 99.7, 52.13, 44.71, and 38.51 kDa, where the 99.70 kDa band corresponds to paramyosin. Additionally, proteins exceeding 200 kDa are identified as myosin heavy chains, while the 52.13, 44.71, and 38.51 kDa bands are likely actin. Acid-soluble proteins have molecular weights mainly distributed at 199.0, 177.33, 106.69, 88.55, and 75.38 kDa, with collagen as the primary component [11]. The traditional Osborne protein extraction method was used to extract mussel protein with four grades, and it was found that the content of alkali-soluble protein in mussels is the highest, followed by water-soluble protein, alcohol-soluble protein and salt-soluble protein [10].

In addition, mussels secrete a highly adhesive protein that enables them to firmly attach to surfaces such as ship hulls, rocks, and pile foundations. This protein is known as mussel foot protein (Mfps). Six types of sticky proteins are involved in the adhesion process, all of which are rich in 3,4-dihydroxyphenylalanine (dopa). Dopa contains catechol functional groups, which confer diverse adhesion capabilities, allowing mussels to form strong bonds on various substrate surfaces. Mfp1 is the most extensively studied sticky protein, with a molecular weight of approximately 110 kDa. It is the largest among all sticky proteins and contains about 10 mol% dopa. Mfp3 and Mfp5 are key functional factors for adhesion, located in the bottom layer of the adhesive disc where they tightly bind to the substrate surface [12]. Mfp3 has the lowest molecular weight among these proteins (6 kDa) and contains around 20 mol% dopa. Mfp5, composed of 74 amino acids, has a low molecular weight of about 9.5 kDa and the highest dopa content of all sticky proteins, at 27 mol%. Mfp2 and Mfp4 account for the highest proportion of all sticky proteins, comprising over 60% by mass. Their molecular weights are 40 kDa and 93 kDa, respectively. However, their dopa contents are relatively low compared to other sticky proteins, approximately 5 mol% in Mfp2 and 4 mol% in Mfp4. Mfp6 has a molecular weight of about 11.6 kDa and a dopa content of 3 mol%, and it is primarily distributed in the bottom layer of the foot disc [13].

2.1.5 Short-Necked Clam

Ruditapes philippinarum, commonly known as the short-necked clam, is one of China's four major cultured shellfish and a key source of aquatic protein. The crude protein content in its soft tissues reaches 61.28% [14]. Among these proteins, salt-soluble proteins are the most abundant in the clam's soft tissues, accounting for 34.83–50.4%, followed by water-soluble proteins (12.55–19.17%), alkali-soluble proteins (17.49–25.06%), and matrix proteins (2.19–10.23%). Protein composition and molecular weight distribution vary across different tissues. In general, the proteins in the foot, adductor muscle, mantle and siphon have similar compositions, with numerous bands and diverse types, including contractile proteins, myosin heavy-chain dimers or polymers, twitch proteins and collagen. In contrast, the gills and visceral mass contain fewer proteins, with molecular weights mainly distributed below 60 kDa. Water-soluble proteins are present in all tissues, which are the foot, adductor muscle, mantle, siphon, gills and visceral mass. For salt-soluble proteins, all tissues except the gills contain characteristic bands corresponding to myosin heavy chain (~200 kDa), paramyosin (~100 kDa), actin or calmodulin (~45 kDa), tropomyosin (~35 kDa), and myosin light chains (< 20 kDa). The gills of *Ruditapes philippinarum* show almost no myostromal protein bands, while in other tissues, myostromal protein bands are mainly distributed above 200 kDa and near 45 kDa. Collagen, the primary component of myostromal proteins, typically consists of three α-chains. Bands above 200 kDa may correspond to β-chains (formed by hydrogen bonding between two 100 kDa α-chains) or γ-chains (formed by hydrogen bonding between three 100 kDa α-chains). Alkali-soluble proteins in the foot, adductor muscle, mantle, and siphon are mainly distributed at 200 kDa, 100 kDa, 45 kDa, and above 200 kDa, while the gills and visceral mass contain almost no alkali-soluble proteins.

The protein content of striated muscle and smooth muscle is also different in the adductor muscle of short-necked clam. Compared with striated muscle, smooth muscle contains a higher content of paramyosin and a lower content of myosin and tropomyosin. The contents of myosin heavy chain, paramyosin, actin, tropomyosin, and myosin light chain in striated muscle and smooth muscle were 19.07% and 12.81%, 27.20% and 7.14%, 23.48% and 22.79%, 23.62% and 18.52%, 6.64% and 3.40%, respectively. Myorod is a specific protein of smooth muscle with a content of 5.34% [5].

2.1.6 Other Marine Shellfish

The edible part of abalone is its gastropod muscle, whose protein is primarily composed of myofibrillar fibers and collagen fibers, accounting for approximately 40–50% and 20–35% of the total protein content, respectively. Regional differences in protein distribution are observed. The middle portion (connected to the shell muscle) has a higher myofibrillar content, while the edge portion is richer in collagen. The muscle fibers of abalone gastropod muscle are mainly striated muscle, where myofibrils exist in a cylindrical form. Key components of abalone myofibrillar proteins, myosin heavy chain, paramyosin, actin, and tropomyosin are primarily distributed around 201 kDa, 96 kDa, 46 kDa, and 38 kDa, respectively. These proteins constitute 21.7%, 35.8%, 27.4%, and 6.6% of total myofibrillar protein. The main collagen type in abalone gastropod muscle is $(\alpha 1)_3$, which can be extracted with its complete triple helix structure preserved using enzyme-assisted dissolution. The relative molecular weight of the abalone collagen α-chain is 175 kDa, and the collagen also contains β-chains and γ-chains.

Clams are a type of marine shellfish that are delicious, rich in protein, and low in fat. In fresh clams, the crude protein content is approximately 10.65%, while the fat content is about 0.31%. Among the proteins, water-soluble protein has the highest content at 44.69%, followed by salt-soluble protein (32.94%) and insoluble protein (16.49%). On electrophoretic bands, the distribution of water-soluble proteins is continuous, mainly concentrated in the range of 25–66 kDa. For salt-soluble proteins, myosin heavy chain, actin, tropomyosin, and paramyosin are distributed around 200 kDa, 44 kDa, 35 kDa, and 100 kDa, respectively. Insoluble proteins, on the other hand, are mainly concentrated in the 44.3–200 kDa range.

2.2 Amino Acid Composition of Marine Shellfish

2.2.1 Overview of Marine Shellfish Amino Acids

The amino acid composition of shellfish is influenced by multiple factors, including season, individual size, feed type, and growing environment. Studies have shown, for instance, that the amino acid content of Pacific lion claw scallops varies with seasons. Glutamic acid and leucine reach their highest levels in summer, while glycine, arginine, and alanine are at their lowest during this period. For other shellfish species, the timing of peak essential amino acid (EAA) content also differs by species. Cockles typically have the highest EAA levels in August and December, variegata cockles in September, and *Sinonovacula constricta* (razor clams) in October. In contrast, oysters generally have relatively low EAA content. At the same time and location, the amino acid content of *Chlamys farreri* (Chinese scallops) of different sizes is inversely proportional to their individual size. Additionally, feed and growing environment impact amino acid composition and content indirectly by regulating the growth and development of shellfish. The quality of shellfish protein is largely determined by the quantity and proportion of essential amino acids. As the basic building blocks of proteins, amino acids are categorized into essential amino acids and nonessential amino acids. Notably, tyrosine and cystine are derived from phenylalanine and methionine, respectively. For adults, the essential amino acids include isoleucine, leucine, lysine, methionine, phenylalanine, threonine, tryptophan, and valine. Infants require two additional essential amino acids, arginine and histidine. These essential amino acids cannot be synthesized by the body and must be obtained from food, making them a key indicator for evaluating nutritional quality. Amino acid profiles are typically assessed using the FAO/WHO scoring model. Sulfur-containing amino acids are often the first limiting amino acids in shellfish and fish, with cystine and methionine being the primary limiting amino acids for most shellfish. Beyond the 20 common amino acids, shellfish are also rich in taurine, which boasts multiple physiological functions such as promoting brain development, protecting the retina, lowering blood pressure, and reducing blood lipids.

Flavor-related amino acids in shellfish mainly include aspartate, glutamic acid, glycine, alanine, serine, and proline. Among these, aspartate and glutamic acid are characteristic umami amino acids, while glycine, alanine, serine, threonine, proline, hydroxyproline, lysine, cysteine, and methionine contribute to sweetness in aquatic products. Shellfish are particularly rich in glycine and alanine, which have strong sweetening properties and thus play a significant role in enhancing the sweet taste of shellfish products. Additionally, shellfish contain branched-chain amino acids (leucine, isoleucine, and valine), which promote protein metabolic synthesis, accelerate muscle growth, and help resist fatigue.

2.2.2 Oyster

Oysters are rich in amino acids, with their water-soluble, salt-soluble, and insoluble proteins all containing 16 common amino acids, which are aspartate, threonine, serine, glutamic acid, glycine, alanine, valine, methionine, isoleucine, leucine, tyrosine, phenylalanine, histidine, lysine, arginine, and proline. Among these three protein fractions, glutamic acid consistently has the highest content, while histidine is the lowest across all fractions. Water-soluble and salt-soluble proteins also have high levels of aspartate and lysine. Insoluble proteins not only contain abundant glutamic acid but are also rich in glycine and proline. Their glycine and proline contents are significantly higher than those in water-soluble and salt-soluble proteins. This is because insoluble proteins are primarily composed of collagen and elastin. Collagen contains approximately 1/3 glycine and 1/4 proline, while elastin has a unique amino acid composition with glycine accounting for 1/3 and proline for 1/2 of its total amino acids. The contents of glutamic acid, leucine and arginine in salt-soluble protein were higher than those in the other two proteins [3].

The contents of essential amino acids in water-soluble protein, salt-soluble protein, and insoluble protein accounted for 40.41%, 41.51%, and 37.87%. The proportion of umami amino acids in proteins was 39.68% in water-soluble protein, 38.02% in salt-soluble protein, and 39.30% in insoluble protein. The branched-chain amino acids in water-soluble protein, salt-soluble protein, and insoluble protein accounted for 17.91%, 19.83%, and 18.54%, respectively. Free umami amino acids are the main components of oyster umami. Oysters contain glutamic acid, glycine, aspartic acid, alanine, arginine, etc. Meanwhile, oysters also contain taurine, which gives oysters a special umami taste [3]. Although there are complete amino acids in oyster protein, the amino acid composition is unbalanced, lacking methionine and tryptophan. The nutrition of oyster protein can be balanced by foods with a high content of methionine and tryptophan. The proportion of essential amino acids to total amino acids in oyster was 40.6%. The ratio of essential amino acids to nonessential amino acids was 0.68. These results were close to the protein model proposed by WHO and FAO (the proportion of essential amino acids to total amino acids should be about 40% and the ratio of essential amino acids to nonessential amino acids should be above 0.77).

2.2.3 Scallop

Scallops are one of China's major aquatic shellfish and are highly popular for their delicious taste. Using an amino acid analyzer, researchers determined the amino acid composition of *Bay scallops* and *Chlamys farreri* from different sea areas. A total of 16 amino acids were detected, along with trace amounts of cystine. Among these, glutamic acid, glycine, and aspartic acid were present in higher concentrations, while proline and histidine were relatively low (Table 2.1). *Bay scallops* sampled from Dalian Bay, Qinhuangdao, Laizhou Bay, Yantai, Weihai, Jiaozhou Bay, and Jiaonan had an average total amino acid content of 54.06%. For *Chlamys farreri* collected from Yantai, Weihai, Jiaozhou Bay, and Jiaonan, the total amino acid content reached 61.23%. Overall, *Chlamys farreri* had significantly higher levels of total amino acids, essential amino acids, and flavor amino acids compared to Bay scallops. According to the FAO/WHO standard model, Bay scallops had an average amino acid score of 82.5–91.5, while *Chlamys farreri* scored 87.5–92.4. Except for methionine, cystine, and valine, all other amino acids scored above 100, indicating that both species have balanced amino acid profiles and comprehensive nutritional value. In *Mizuhopecten yessoensis*, essential amino acids accounted for 36.52% of total amino acids, close to the 40% standard set by FAO/WHO. This species also

Table 2.1 Amino acid composition of oyster and scallop (g/100 g) [3, 4, 14, 15]

	Oyster			Scallop			
Amino acid	Water-soluble protein	Salt-soluble protein	Insoluble protein	*Bay scallops*	*Chlamys farreri*	*Mizuhopecten yessoensis*	Scallop-isolated protein
Asp	11.83	10.99	10.93	5.46	6.40	1.48	11.42
Thr	4.54	4.49	4.52	2.36	2.67	0.64	3.94
Ser	3.77	4.10	4.25	2.35	2.72	0.6	3.36
Glu	14.96	16.64	14.92	7.89	9.35	2.51	17.89
Gly	6.33	4.05	7.99	7.79	7.48	2.34	3.57
Ala	6.46	6.33	5.44	3.10	3.43	0.95	6.05
Val	5.69	5.29	5.93	2.40	2.65	0.67	4.87
Met	3.32	3.29	3.31	1.51	1.71	0.49	2.97
Ile	5.50	5.48	5.13	2.23	2.61	0.73	4.87
Leu	6.72	9.06	7.48	3.90	4.64	1.19	9.02
Tyr	3.13	3.63	4.17	1.57	1.84	0.55	3.42
Phe	6.14	3.88	4.11	1.93	2.26	0.7	4.55
His	3.07	1.38	1.68	1.14	1.20	0.37	1.82
Lys	8.50	10.02	7.39	3.77	4.44	1.27	8.88
Arg	6.07	8.92	7.64	4.70	5.74	1.35	8.59
Pro	3.97	2.45	5.11	1.19	1.26	0.64	2.94
Cys	–	–	–	–	–	0.10	0.35
Trp	–	–	–	–	–	–	1.53

contained taurine at 7.33 mg/g, while *Chlamys farreri* had a slightly higher taurine content of 7.55 mg/g.

In scallop protein isolates extracted using the pH adjustment method, glutamic acid and aspartic acid are the most abundant, with significant levels of leucine, lysine, and arginine also present (Table 2.1). The essential amino acid (EAA) content of these isolates is approximately 46.22%, showing no significant difference from the EAA content of protein isolates from clams and abalones. According to recommendations from FAO/WHO/UNU, the essential amino acid profile of scallop protein isolates meets the amino acid requirements for both adults and infants. Tryptophan is the first limiting amino acid in scallop protein isolates, followed by methionine, cysteine, and histidine. Additionally, the branched-chain amino acid (BCAA) content of scallop protein isolates is about 18.76%, slightly lower than that of protein isolates from clams and abalones [15].

2.2.4 Mussel

Mussel proteins contain a complete and abundant range of amino acids, including all amino acids required by animals. Notably, their content of the eight essential amino acids for humans is higher than that of milk, chicken, duck, and other animal meats, making mussel protein a high-quality protein source [11]. In *Perna viridis* (green mussels), glutamic acid, glycine, and aspartic acid are the most abundant amino acids, with significant levels of lysine, threonine, and isoleucine also present. Essential amino acids account for 33.2% of the amino acids in the soft tissues of *Perna viridis*, a proportion similar to that of *Bay scallops*, *Chlamys farreri*, *Mytilus edulis* (blue mussels), and *Ruditapes philippinarum* (short-necked clams). Based on the amino acid pattern recommended by FAO/WHO, *Perna viridis* has an amino acid score of 81, indicating high nutritional value. In protein isolates from *Mytilus unguiculatus* (hooked mussels), glutamic acid and aspartic acid are the most abundant. Essential amino acids make up approximately 36% of these isolates, with particularly high levels of lysine, leucine, phenylalanine, threonine, and valine [16]. Among the water-soluble, salt-soluble, alcohol-soluble, and alkali-soluble proteins of *Perna viridis*, all contain high levels of glutamic acid, aspartic acid, lysine, and serine. Beyond water-soluble proteins, the other three fractions (salt-soluble, alcohol-soluble, and alkali-soluble) also have high contents of leucine, valine, threonine, and tyrosine. Additionally, alcohol-soluble proteins have significantly higher levels of methionine and cysteine than other protein fractions, while alkali-soluble proteins are richer in phenylalanine and threonine compared to others (Table 2.2) [10]. The ratio of essential to nonessential amino acids in total *Perna viridis* protein is 0.66, higher than the reference standard proposed by WHO/FAO. However, this ratio is exceptionally low in water-soluble proteins (0.29). In contrast, the ratios in salt-soluble, alcohol-soluble, and alkali-soluble proteins are either higher than or close to the reference standard [10]. Umami-characteristic amino acids (glutamic acid and aspartic acid) and sweet-characteristic amino acids (glycine and alanine)

Table 2.2 Amino acid composition of mussel (g/100 g) [10, 16]

Amino acid	*Perna viridis*	*Mytilus unguiculatus*	*Mytilus edulis*				
			Mytilus edulis protein	Water-soluble protein	Salt-soluble protein	Alcohol-soluble protein	Alkali-soluble protein
Asp	9.62	12.79	11.68	16.32	10.89	10.33	11.65
Thr	3.69	4.87	5.70	3.60	5.62	5.22	6.13
Ser	3.00	4.36	4.95	4.62	4.73	5.34	4.98
Glu	13.18	14.58	14.11	20.91	12.37	12.80	13.56
Gly	9.70	4.03	6.16	12.80	4.58	5.08	4.54
Ala	5.32	4.26	4.79	3.40	3.93	3.09	4.43
Val	4.55	4.47	4.80	2.74	5.92	6.78	5.23
Met	2.01	2.46	2.23	2.15	3.65	7.51	2.91
Ile	4.24	4.84	4.23	1.33	3.91	2.76	4.62
Leu	6.51	6.35	7.09	2.42	7.16	4.79	8.16
Tyr	2.65	4.30	3.96	1.68	4.81	5.33	4.84
Phe	3.67	5.03	4.93	1.24	5.22	1.84	6.03
His	1.54	2.08	2.28	1.83	2.38	1.71	2.44
Lys	6.19	6.75	7.95	6.40	8.07	5.07	7.57
Arg	6.62	7.81	6.84	9.87	5.28	3.23	5.69
Pro	3.73	3.25	4.53	1.65	3.27	2.71	4.78
Cys	0.89	2.95	2.34	2.77	5.73	12.13	1.2

together account for 28.7% of the total amino acids in mussels. The synergistic effect of these flavor amino acids contributes to the umami and sweet taste of *Mytilus edulis*.

In addition, the taurine of mussels is also rich. The taurine content of *Mytilus edulis* was as high as 36 mg/g and that of *Perna viridis* was 802 mg/100 g, which was slightly lower than that of *Pinctada martensii* and oyster, and higher than that of other shellfish.

2.2.5 *Short-Necked Clam*

The soft tissues of short-necked clams contain a complete range of amino acids, with 18 amino acids detected via high-performance liquid chromatography (HPLC). Among these, glutamic acid and aspartic acid content reaches 8.39% and 4.88%, respectively, while cystine content is relatively low at 0.44%. In terms of classification, essential amino acids account for 21.58%, semi-essential amino acids for 6.82%, and nonessential amino acids for 24.46% of the total. Notably, essential amino acids make up 40.82% of total amino acids, aligning with the ideal standard of 40% recommended by FAO/WHO, confirming that the protein in short-necked clam soft tissues is of high quality. Based on amino acid scores, methionine and cystine are the first limiting amino acids, followed by isoleucine as the second limiting amino acid. From a flavor perspective, the combined content of key taste-related amino acids, glutamic acid, aspartic acid, alanine, and glycine reaches 18.89%. Specifically, glycine and alanine content are 2.49% and 3.13%, respectively, which enhances the delicious umami and sweet notes of short-necked clams.

Amino acid composition varies between fresh short-necked clams, boiled clams, and their primary, secondary, and tertiary boiling solutions. While 18 amino acids are detected in both fresh and boiled clams, only 16 are found in the boiling solutions, with methionine and cysteine absent. The ratio of essential amino acids to total amino acids is 35.34% in fresh clams, 35.79% in boiled clams, and 23.38%, 22.74%, and 22.16% in the primary, secondary, and tertiary boiling solutions, respectively.

Based on the amino acid scoring criteria recommended by FAO/WHO, all amino acids in both fresh and cooked short-necked clams scored over 90, except for methionine, meaning they can meet human nutritional needs. Specifically, methionine scores in fresh and cooked clams were only 37.39 and 27.96, respectively. In contrast, among the primary, secondary, and tertiary boiling solutions of short-necked clams, only threonine and lysine meet human requirements. For these boiling solutions, methionine is the first limiting amino acid, while phenylalanine and tyrosine are the second limiting amino acids. Notably, the total content of flavor amino acids in cooked clams and their boiling solutions is higher than in fresh clams. However, the content of umami amino acids in the boiling solutions is lower than that in fresh clams (Table 2.3) [17].

2.2.6 *Other Marine Shellfish*

The total amino acid content of abalone muscle is 49.63 g/100 g. Among these amino acids, glutamic acid is the most abundant at 8.49 g/100 g, while tryptophan is the lowest at 0.48 g/100 g. In addition to glutamic acid, arginine, aspartic acid, glycine, and leucine are also present in high amounts. In abalone muscle proteins, glutamic acid remains the most abundant amino acid in both water-soluble and salt-soluble fractions, whereas hydroxyproline is the lowest in these fractions. Since insoluble proteins are primarily composed of collagen, they have the highest glycine content and are also rich in proline and hydroxyproline. Although abalone muscle and its protein fractions all contain the eight essential amino acids required by humans, only the water-soluble proteins meet the evaluation criteria set by FAO/WHO. The flavor amino acid content in abalone muscle accounts for 62.35% of total amino acids. This proportion is close to that of salt-soluble proteins, higher than that of water-soluble proteins (50.63%), but lower than that of insoluble proteins (73.81%). Flavor amino acids in abalone muscle are mainly concentrated in salt-soluble and insoluble proteins. From a nutritional perspective, abalone water-soluble proteins are closer to the ideal protein pattern, while salt-soluble and insoluble proteins make greater contributions to abalone's flavor.

Table 2.3 Amino acid composition of short-necked clam and its boiled solution (g/100 g) [17]

Amino acid	Crude protein	Dry sample	Fresh sample	Boiled short-necked clam	Primary boiling solution	Secondary boiling solution	Tertiary boiling solution
Asp	8.77	4.88	10.68	10.67	13.58	13.57	13.44
Thr	5.26	2.93	4.08	4.61	3.94	3.76	3.82
Ser	2.01	2.01	3.43	3.69	3.58	3.45	3.38
Glu	15.07	8.39	12.57	12.79	11.28	11.44	11.53
Gly	4.47	2.49	6.58	5.94	11.67	12.09	12.08
Cys	0.79	0.44	0.24	0.21	–	–	–
Trp	0.88	0.49	1.29	1.10	2.09	1.86	1.82
Ala	5.62	3.13	6.04	5.41	8.18	8.43	8.25
Val	6.09	3.39	5.11	5.14	3.18	2.96	2.17
Met	2.25	1.25	1.31	0.98	–	–	–
Ile	3.61	2.01	4.28	4.41	1.72	1.71	1.72
Leu	7.71	4.29	6.46	6.66	2.76	2.74	2.76
Tyr	3.63	2.02	2.07	2.07	0.45	0.45	0.49
Phe	2.93	1.63	3.40	3.58	1.38	1.26	1.32
His	4.85	2.70	14.01	14.20	20.35	20.46	21.20
Lys	5.62	3.13	9.42	9.32	8.33	8.44	8.56
Arg	7.40	4.12	6.16	6.40	5.00	5.05	5.11
Pro	6.40	3.56	2.88	2.86	2.52	2.32	2.36

Clam proteins, including their water-soluble, salt-soluble, and insoluble fractions, contain a total of 17 amino acids. Among these, glutamic acid is the most abundant across both whole clams and the three protein components, accounting for 15.74% (whole clams), 14.60% (water-soluble proteins), 19.59% (salt-soluble proteins), and 15.05% (insoluble proteins), respectively. Notably, insoluble proteins also have a high glycine content (11.35%), which aligns with the characteristic amino acid profile of collagen. In terms of essential amino acids, their contents in whole clams and the three protein fractions are 37.30%, 36.57%, 37.91%, and 32.92% respectively, with whole clams and salt-soluble proteins showing values closer to the ideal FAO/WHO model. Additionally, water-soluble and insoluble proteins are rich in flavor amino acids, with their contents reaching 51.55% and 52.94%, respectively (Table 2.4) [18].

Seventeen common amino acids were detected in the muscles of *Ruditapes philippinarum*, *Saxidomus purpurata*, *Mizuhopecten yessoensis*, *Scapharca broughtonii*, *Scapharca subcrenata*, *Haliotis discus hannai ino*, *Rapana venosa*, and *Octopus variabilis sasaki*. Among them, the contents of glutamic acid, alanine, aspartate, and glycine were higher. The essential amino acid index was the highest in *Scapharca broughtonii*, and the lowest in *Ruditapes philippinarum*. The first limiting amino acid was valine in all the samples except for *Scapharca subcrenata* [4].

Table 2.4 Amino acid composition of abalone and clam (g/100 g) [18]

Amino acid	Abalone				Clam			
	Muscle	Water-soluble protein	Salt-soluble protein	Insoluble protein	Clam	Water-soluble protein	Salt-soluble protein	Insoluble protein
Asp	4.93	3.45	12.30	7.61	10.11	10.44	12.06	10.86
Thr	2.33	1.52	4.72	2.31	4.59	4.56	4.46	4.35
Ser	2.30	1.46	4.87	4.92	4.04	3.66	4.36	4.48
Glu	8.49	3.99	20.85	13.61	15.74	14.60	19.59	15.05
Gly	4.44	1.48	3.48	19.36	6.60	7.34	3.05	11.35
Ala	2.80	1.70	6.60	6.57	8.97	11.67	6.90	4.84
Val	2.06	1.73	5.00	2.17	4.57	4.84	4.27	4.01
Met	1.17	0.75	3.06	1.68	2.57	2.19	2.31	2.80
Ile	1.99	1.53	5.04	1.42	4.46	4.23	4.30	3.97
Leu	3.63	2.24	8.45	2.11	7.76	6.53	9.98	6.67
Tyr	1.73	1.30	3.89	2.05	3.61	3.00	3.35	4.38
Phe	1.59	1.49	3.71	1.60	3.96	4.21	3.03	3.95
His	0.87	1.04	1.63	0.11	1.89	2.29	1.43	1.77
Lys	1.31	2.30	1.46	0.78	7.28	7.51	8.03	5.05
Arg	6.24	2.30	10.74	9.10	7.89	6.60	9.02	7.98
Pro	1.74	1.10	4.16	6.63	3.85	3.86	2.34	6.36
Try	0.48	0.32	0.48	0.46	2.11	2.50	1.52	2.13
Cys	0.68	0.61	0.79	3.01	–	–	–	–

2.3 The Stability of Marine Shellfish Protein

Heat treatment is a common way to process aquatic products, and heating can cause changes in protein structure and functional properties. Shellfish proteins usually have high thermal stability. Almost no obvious denaturation of proteins in oysters, scallops, and mussels are observed below 40 °C, and the thermal denaturation temperature of actin is usually higher than that of myosin.

The β-turn content of oyster protein obtained by water extraction and acid precipitation decreased with the increase of heating temperature, the random coil content increased, and the protein hydrophobic coefficient increased, indicating that oyster protein unfolded and exposed more hydrophobic groups. The turbidity, solubility, surface hydrophobicity, α-helix content, and total sulfhydryl content of myofibrillar protein in oyster adductor muscle had no significant changes in the temperature range of 20–40 °C. The solubility and surface hydrophobicity changed the most at the temperature range of 40–50 °C, and the turbidity changed the most at 46 °C [19]. The thermal denaturation temperature of oyster paramyosin was 51.7 ± 0.2 °C. After heating at 80 °C, the α-helix content decreased. The α-helix structure content increased when the temperature was reduced to 20 °C, but it could not return to the original value, indicating that part of oyster paramyosin underwent irreversible thermal denaturation after heating. The monomer content on the

SDS-PAGE electrophoresis strip decreased, and large molecular weight polymers appeared when oyster paramyosin was heated to 80 °C [2]. Differential scanning calorimetry (DSC) was used to measure the thermal denaturation temperature of the water-soluble protein at 60 °C, and the thermal denaturation temperature of myosin and actin in the salt-soluble protein were 48.1 °C and 95.3 °C, respectively. On the DSC curve of oyster insoluble protein, there was a heat absorption peak at 118.9 °C [3].

The DSC spectra of the striated muscle and smooth muscle of *Zygochlamys patagonica* showed two transformations, T_{max} 55.0, 79.2 °C and T_{max} 54.7, 78.7 °C, respectively. The DSC spectra of myofibril and actomyosin are similar to those corresponding to their respective entire muscles. pH and ionic strength affected the thermal stability of scallop muscles. The thermal stability of the whole scallop muscle decreased with the increase of pH and ionic strength. However, when the pH increased from 5.0 to 8.0, the enthalpy of degeneration of the whole striated muscle decreased significantly. A significant reduction in the sum of ΔH, as well as the peak I of ΔH, was also observed in the DSC of smooth muscle at pH 8.0. When the ionic strength increased from 0.05 to 0.5, the ΔH sum and the ΔH peak I of both muscles were significantly decreased. The striated muscle of *Zygochlamys patagonica* was generally more susceptible to change in the chemical environment than smooth muscle [6]. The thermal stability of the adductor protein of *Mizuhopecten yessoensis* is affected by heating temperature and heating time. After the adductor muscle was treated at 60 °C, 80 °C, and 100 °C, the actomyosin peptide chain of the adductor muscle of the *Mizuhopecten yessoensis* was uncoiled, and the protein irregularly accumulated. With the increase of heating time, the turbidity of the protein solution increased, the surface hydrophobicity increased, and the content of active -SH and α-helix decreased. The higher temperature of heat treatment, the phenomenon was also obvious [20]. There was no significant changes in Ca^{2+}-ATPase activity of myofibrillar protein after 30 °C and 35 °C heating for 30 min. The activity began to decline at 40 °C, and the activity of Ca^{2+}-ATPase decreased sharply at 45 °C. The activity of Ca^{2+}-ATPase in striated muscle and smooth muscle was all inactivated after heating at 50 °C for 10 min. In addition, there were seasonal differences in the thermal stability of striated muscle and smooth muscle. The deactivation rate of striated muscle was higher than that of smooth muscle in spring, and there was little difference in summer, autumn, and winter. On the whole, the muscle protein of *Mizuhopecten yessoensis* had the worst thermal stability in spring [21].

The thermal denaturation temperature of salt-soluble protein in mussels was 46.5 °C, among which myosin had the worst thermal stability at 40–60 °C, actin had the strongest thermal stability, and denaturation began at 71 °C [22]. The thermal stability of mussel paramyosin was better than that of *Portuguese oyster* and *Haliotis discus hannai ino*, and its thermal denaturation temperature was 56.3 ± 0.2 °C [2]. The paramyosin of *Perna viridis* was reversibly denatured during heating, and the α-helix decreased after heating at 90 °C. When the temperature was reduced to 20 °C, the α-helix returned to the original value. The protein bands of *Perna viridis* paramyosin showed no significant changes after heating at 30–100 °C.

The temperature of clam protein denaturation was relatively low. There are two absorption peaks in the DSC curve of the salt-soluble protein of clam. The DSC curves of salt-soluble protein and insoluble protein were relatively smooth, and the heat absorption peaks were not obvious. The denaturation temperature of clam was 49.5 °C, and the temperature of water-soluble protein was the lowest, 38.8 °C. Since salt-soluble protein contained myosin and actin, the thermal stability of actin was higher than that of myosin. The two absorption peaks of 41.7 °C and 60.9 °C on the DSC curve of salt-soluble protein represented the thermal denaturation temperatures of myosin and actin. The thermal denaturation temperature of insoluble protein was 43.2 °C. The thermal denaturation temperature of clam-isolated protein was 63.6 °C, higher than that of scallop (57.0 °C) and abalone isolated protein (61.6 °C) [15].

The turbidity of the myofibrillar protein solution of *Haliotis discus hannai ino* remained unchanged at 30–40 °C but increased significantly at 40–50 °C. The turbidity of the solution was 1.0 at 50 °C. As the temperature increased to 90 °C, the turbidity rose slowly. Similarly, the solubility of abalone gastropod myofibrillar protein did not change significantly at 30–40 °C, but decreased sharply at 40–50 °C, indicating that abalone gastropod myofibrillar protein rapidly denatured at this temperature. When the temperature rose to 90 °C, the solubility decreased slowly, indicating that the undenatured protein was slowly denaturing. The thermal denaturation temperature of *Haliotis discus hannai ino* paramyosin was 52.5 ± 0.2 °C. After heating at 80 °C, the characteristic peak of the α-helix structure was very small. When the temperature was restored to 20 °C, the α-helix structure returned to the original value. The secondary structure of paramyosin was reversible from heating to cooling [2]. The thermal stability of enzyme-soluble collagen of abalone muscle was lower than that of acid-soluble collagen. The thermal denaturation temperature of acid-soluble collagen was 34.2 °C. The thermal denaturation temperature of enzyme-soluble collagen decreased with the increase of enzyme concentration.

pH can affect the charge distribution of the amino acid side chain, enhance or weaken the interaction between protein molecules, and change the state of the protein. Therefore, the physicochemical properties of protein solution are affected by pH. In general, shellfish protein has the lowest solubility at the isoelectric point and increase solubility away from the isoelectric point. Shellfish protein is easily dissolved under alkaline conditions and precipitated under acidic conditions. The Ca^{2+}-ATPase activity in myofibrillar protein is the most stable under neutral conditions.

The content of oyster protein extracted from Dalian Bay increased first and then decreased in the range of pH 9–13 and reached the peak at pH 12. Therefore, the optimal alkali-soluble pH of Dalian Bay oyster protein was 12. In the range of pH 3.2–6.5, the content of oyster protein first decreased and then increased with the increase of pH, and reached the lowest value at pH 4.0. The optimal acid precipitation pH of Dalian Bay oyster protein was 4.0 [23]. The solubility of the water-soluble protein of oyster was higher than that of salt-soluble protein. The nitrogen solubility index of water-soluble protein and salt-soluble protein was the lowest near pH 4 and 6, respectively. The isoelectric points of the two proteins were near pH 4 and 6, respectively. The relationship between water-holding capacity and pH of oyster protein was the same as that of solubility. The water-holding capacity of oyster protein was low near the isoelectric point and increased in the range of pH 6–10. The foamability of oyster protein was low near the isoelectric point. When deviated from the isoelectric point, oyster protein had good foamability and stability. The changing trend of emulsification of oyster protein with pH was similar to that of solubility [3]. The accumulation and precipitation of oyster paramyosin occurred when the pH was less than 6, but oyster paramyosin was stable under neutral and alkaline conditions [2].

The myosin Ca^{2+}-ATPase activity in the adductor muscle of *Chlamys farreri* was the most stable under neutral conditions [24]. The isoelectric point of the adductor muscle and the coated myofibrillar protein of the *Mizuhopecten yessoensis* is near pH 5. The solubility of the two myofibrillar proteins increased rapidly when away from the isoelectric point [25]. The two myofibrillar proteins had the best solubility at pH 2 and 11, respectively. The Ca^{2+}-ATPase activity of the two myofibrillar proteins was also the most stable under neutral conditions [6]. The physical, chemical, and heat-induced gel properties of *Mizuhopecten yessoensis*is actomyosin were also affected by pH. When the pH was low, the turbidity and surface hydrophobicity of actomyosin solution were higher, and the α-helix content was lower. At the same temperature, the turbidity and surface hydrophobicity of the solution decreased with the pH increased from 5.6 to 8.0. The variation trend of α-helix content was opposite to that of turbidity and surface hydrophobicity. Actomyosin of scallops was more sensitive under acidic conditions than alkaline conditions, and the changes in turbidity and surface hydrophobicity were always consistent. Scallop actomyosin heat-induced gel showed better water-holding capacity at higher pH [26].

Mytilus unguiculatus isolated protein had good solubility in pH < 3 or pH > 5, and the solubility was low at pH 3–5. The isolated protein of *Mytilus unguiculatus* had good foaming properties under acidic and alkaline conditions, and the foam stability was the best under neutral conditions [16]. *Mytilus edulis* protein had low solubility in the pH range of 3.5–4.5, below 5%. In the pH range of 5–10, the solubility of *Mytilus edulis* protein gradually increased with the increase of pH, and reached 64% at pH 10. Similarly, the solubility of *Mytilus edulis* protein increased as the pH dropped from 3.0 to 2.0 [10]. Under neutral and alkaline conditions, paramyosin of *Perna viridis* maintained good stability. Under acidic conditions, paramyosin of *Perna viridis* accumulated and precipitated [2]. The pH also affected the molecular size and mussel hydrolysate stability. The protein content of the enzymolysis polypeptide solution of mussels was the highest at pH 8.0. The protein content was below 50 μg/mL at pH 2.0–3.0. The isoelectric point of protein in the enzymolysis solution was about 5. The protein in the enzymolysis solution of mussels was more stable under alkaline conditions than acidic conditions [27].

The isoelectric point of the protomyosin of the *Ruditapes philippinarum* was about 5.1. The tropomyosin of the *Ruditapes philippinarum* was dissolved in the pH 1.0–11.0 buffer at room temperature for 2 h, the electrophoresis bands of tropomyosin did not change significantly at pH 1.0–7.0 but dispersed at pH 8.0–11.0. In the range of pH 2.0–11.0, the content of α-helix in the secondary structure of *Ruditapes philippinarum* increased with the increase of pH, and the content of random curl gradually decreased. The pH also affected the surface hydrophobicity of *Ruditapes philippinarum* tropomyosin. In the range of pH 2.0–7.0, the surface hydrophobicity gradually decreased with the increase of pH. There were no significant differences in the hydrophobicity at pH 7.0–11.0. The UV absorption peak of tropomyosin was about 270 nm under the neutral conditions. The exposure of tyrosine and tryptophan caused the extension of protein structure under the acidic environment, and the UV absorption peak of tropomyosin was slightly redshifted [28].

The optimal pH for alkaline extraction and acid precipitation of clam and abalone were 12 and 5.1, respectively. The dissolution curves of the two proteins were parabolic in the range of pH 2.0–12.0 [15]. The solubility of abalone gastropod myofibrillar protein was low at the pH < 5.5. The solubility increased sharply in the range of pH 5.5–6.0. When pH > 6.5, there was no significant changes in solubility. The turbidity of the abalone gastropod myofibrillar protein solution was also affected by pH. The turbidity was large and fluctuated at pH 4.0, 4.5, and 5.0. Abalone gastropod myofibrillar protein was prone to aggregation under acidic conditions. There was almost no aggregation under neutral and alkaline conditions. The muscle paramyosin of *Haliotis discus hannai ino* is an acidic protein, which can maintain good stability in the pH range of 6.0–11.0. There was obvious aggregation at pH 5.0 and precipitation. As the pH decreased to 3.0–4.0, almost all paramyosin precipitated [2]. The isoelectric point of enzyme-soluble collagen was 5.17, and the foaming property was 110% in the range of pH 3.0–3.5, but the foam stability was poor.

2.4 The Ion-Binding Properties of Marine Shellfish Protein

Some shellfish also contain special proteins with metal ion-binding properties. Oysters, for instance, are rich in glutamic acid, leucine, arginine, and aspartic acid, amino acids that exhibit strong affinity for metal binding. From oyster protein hydrolysates, zinc ion-binding peptides can be isolated and purified. The interaction between zinc and these oyster peptides primarily occurs through amino nitrogen atoms and carboxyl oxygen atoms [29]. Ferritin, a universal iron storage protein present in all living organisms, can store large amounts of soluble nontoxic iron. Structurally, it consists of a 12 nm shell and an 8 nm diameter iron core. Its inner chamber serves as a reaction chamber with a well-defined size and the capacity to synthesize nanoparticles. Beyond storing and transporting iron, ferritin can also sequester nutrients like calcium, zinc, vitamins, and other health-beneficial organic substances under appropriate conditions. The ferritin gene GF1 was cloned by extracting RNA from oyster viscera, followed by heterologous expression to obtain oyster ferritin. Purified oyster ferritin consists of a single subunit with a molecular weight of 19,958 Da, and its electrophoretic band corresponds to a molecular weight of approximately 480 kDa [30]. In addition, a 20 kDa protein purified from Pacific oysters and Portuguese oysters has been identified as sarcoplasmic calcium-binding protein, a potential new sensitizer in oysters [31].

Metallothioneins (MTs) play a key role in the biochemical detoxification of potentially toxic metals. These well-known low-molecular-weight (6–7 kDa) cytoplasmic metal-binding proteins are ubiquitous in eukaryotes, characterized by a high proportion of cysteine residues (approximately 30%) arranged in globular domains or clusters. They exhibit varying metal ion-binding affinities, with a preference order of zinc > cadmium > copper > silver > mercury. Their key biological roles include regulating homeostasis of essential metals like zinc and copper, as well as detoxifying harmful heavy metals (e.g., cadmium, mercury) through chelation [32]. Studies have investigated how metal exposure affects MT synthesis and lipid peroxidation in two bivalve mollusks (Pacific oysters and *Mytilus edulis*). After 4 days of metal exposure, cadmium and mercury accumulated in the gills and digestive glands, yet total protein levels showed no significant change. After 21 days, however, metals bioaccumulated in the gills and digestive glands of both species. Total protein concentrations decreased in oyster gills and mussel digestive glands, while MT levels in the gills of both mollusks increased. Metallothioneins thus play a critical role in metal metabolism, particularly in detoxification, by acting as chelators for excess cellular metals. Metal exposure in various mollusks consistently induces the production of these low-molecular-weight, cysteine-rich proteins [33].

Heavy metal accumulation in *Mizuhopecten yessoensis* (Yesso scallops) is also linked to intracellular metal-binding proteins. Cadmium accumulates at higher levels than copper and lead, with most accumulated metals concentrated in the digestive glands. Three proteins with molecular weights of approximately 28, 37, and 42 kDa were isolated from these digestive glands. Amino acid sequence analysis revealed high similarity to metallothioneins and ion transporters, suggesting their involvement in metal accumulation and detoxification mechanisms in *Mizuhopecten yessoensis* [34].

2.5 Summary

As aquatic products rich in protein, shellfish boast high nutritional value. Their proteins contain a complete range of amino acids, with abundant aspartic acid and glutamic acid being key contributors to the characteristic umami taste of shellfish. Additionally, shellfish contain specialized ion-binding proteins, such as zinc-binding proteins, ferritin, and metallothioneins, which endow their proteins with unique functional properties. By leveraging modern advanced food processing technologies, deep processing of shellfish and the development of diversified products represent effective strategies to fully utilize shellfish resources.

References

1. FAO. The state of world fisheries and aquaculture 2019. Rome: Food and Agriculture Organization of the United Nations; 2019.
2. Tanaka H, Ishimaru S, Nagatsuka Y, Ohashi K. Smooth muscle-like Ca^{2+}-regulation of actin–myosin interaction in adult jellyfish striated muscle. Sci Rep. 2018;8(1):7776–87.
3. Pascual M, Pla M. Changes in collagen, texture and sensory properties of meat when selecting rabbits for growth rate. Meat Sci. 2008;78(4):375–80.
4. Epstein HF, Miller DM 3rd, Ortiz I, Berliner GC. Myosin and paramyosin are organized about a newly identified core structure. J Cell Biol. 1985;100(3):904–15.
5. Zhang L, Liu J, Tian Y, Liu J, Wu Z, Wang W. Composition and distribution of nitrogenous compounds in soft body of *Ruditapes philippinarum*. Food Sci. 2015;36(24):95–100.
6. Paredi ME, Tomas MC, Crupkin M. Thermal denaturation of myofibrillar proteins of striated and smooth adductor muscles of scallop (*Zygochlamys patagonica*): a differential scanning calorimetric study. J Agric Food Chem. 2002;50(4):830–4.
7. Zhang J, Zheng H, Zhang C, Hao J, Zhang J, Zhang J. The separation and composition of oyster protein. Food Ferment Ind. 2013;39(9):195–9.
8. Song Y, Zhang Q, Zhou Y, Liu H, Zheng Y, Tian Y, Liu J. Protein distribution and physicochemical properties in striated muscle and smooth muscle of Patinopecten yessoensis. J Fish China. 2017;41(11):1798–805.
9. Xin C, Liu JR, Cai QF, Zhang CH, Cao MJ. Primary processing parameters and protein compositions in three commercial scallop species. Fish Sci. 2012;31(9):535–9.
10. Cushman DW, Cheung HS, Sabo EF, Ondetti MA. Development and design of specific inhibitors of angiotensin-converting enzyme. Am J Cardiol. 1982;49(6):1390–4.
11. Qiao M, Tu M, Wang Z, Mao F, Chen H, Qin L, Du M. Identification and antithrombotic activity of peptides from blue mussel (*Mytilus edulis*) protein. Int J Mol Sci. 2018;19(1):138.
12. Ai Y, Wei Y, Nie J, Yang D. Study on the synthesis and properties of mussel mimetic poly(*Ethylene glycol*) bioadhesive. J Photochem Photobiol B Biol. 2013;120:183–90.
13. Xiong X, Liu Y, Shi F, Zhang G, Weng J, Qu S. Enhanced adhesion of mussel-inspired adhesive through manipulating contents of dopamine methacrylamide and molecular weight of polymer. J Bionic Eng. 2018;15(3):461–70.
14. Wu Y, Liang J, Yan X, Zhao L, Yang F. Analysis of the nutritional components of manila clam Ruditapes philippinarum. Acta Nutr Sin. 2012;34(4):409–10.
15. Xue G, Zhang K, Zheng Y, Zheng H, Zhou C, Gao J, Qin X, Zhang C. Extraction of three shellfish protein isolates by isoelectric solubilisation/precipitation and their composition and characteristics analysis. Food Ferment Ind. 2018;44(10):145–51.
16. Zhang Q, Marius N, Zhang L, Li D. Study on extraction, amino acid composition and physicochemical properties of Mytilus coruscus protein isolate. Sci Technol Food Ind. 2012;33(24):154–7.
17. Zhu M, Hao S, Qin L, Li D, Xu X, Dong L, Du M. Analysis of nutritional composition and flavor compounds in boiled clam liquid. Sci Technol Food Ind. 2017;38(3):57–63.
18. Tang X, Zheng H, Zhang C, Hao J, Zhang J. Protein composition analysis and molecular weight distribution of Meretrix lusoria. Sci Technol Food Ind. 2015;36(22):362–6.
19. Chen Z, Zhu B, Li D, Jiang P, Zhao X, Deng L. Physiochemical changes of myofibrillar protein from oyster adductor muscle during heat treatment. Food Ferment Ind. 2012;38(7):53–7.
20. Wang J, Zhu B, Dong X, Chen X, Zheng J. Effect of thermal treatment on biochemical properties of actomyosin from adductor muscles of scallop. Food Ferment Ind. 2012;38(2):22–6.
21. Zhang Q, Tian Y, Jiang M, Liu J. Seasonal variation of myofibrillar protein thermal stability of scallop (*Patinopecten yessoensis*). J Fish China. 2020;44(11):1883–92.
22. Qiao M, Liu H, Fan F, Tu M, Yu C, Du M. Characterization of salt-soluble protein from mytilus edulis and enzymatic preparation of ACE inhibitory peptides. Food Sci. 2018;39(22):51–6.
23. Yan-Rong J, Ya-Fei Z, Xiao-Ying Q, Dan-Ni W, Mao-Hong T, Hui Z. Analysis of oyster protein extracted by isoelectric precipitation. J Fish Res. 2019;41(2):106–12.

24. Yokomoto K, Nishita K. Heat denaturation of akazara striated myosin. Bull Jpn Soc Sci Fish. 1987;53(3):451–6.
25. Liang S, Liu J, Ma Y, Wu Z, Yan R, Li F. Isolation and functional properties of roteins from patinopecten yessoensis mantle. Food Sci. 2014;35(7):12–6.
26. Dong XP, Ma LL, Zheng J, Wang JT, Wu Q, Song S, Zhou DY. Effect of pH on the physicochemical and heat-induced gel properties of scallop Patinopecten yessoensis actomyosin. Fish Sci. 2014;80(5):1073–82.
27. Mao F, Yi J, Qiao M, Wang Z, Qin L, Du M. Influence factors of stability of the enzymatic system of proteins from mytilus edulis and its mechanism. J Chin Inst Food Sci Technol. 2019;19(4):100–8.
28. Lin HX, Li ZX, Lin H, Song YN, Lv LT, Hao ZN. Effect of pH shifts on IgE-binding capacity and conformational structure of tropomyosin from short-neck clam (*Ruditapes philippinarum*). Food Chem. 2015;188:248–55.
29. Chen D, Liu ZY, Huang WQ, Zhao YH, Dong SY, Zeng MY. Purification and characterisation of a zinc-binding peptide from oyster protein hydrolysate. J Funct Foods. 2013;5(2):689–97.
30. Li H, Tan XY, Xia XY, Zang JC, Wang ZY, Du M. Thermal treatment modified the physicochemical properties of recombinant oyster (*Crassostrea gigas*) ferritin. Food Chem. 2020;314:126210.
31. Han TJ, Liu M, Huan F, Li MS, Xia F, Chen YY, Chen GX, Cao MJ, Liu GM. Identification and cross-reactivity analysis of sarcoplasmic-calcium-binding protein: a novel allergen in *Crassostrea angulata*. J Agric Food Chem. 2020;68(18):5221–31.
32. Bernal-Hernández YY, Medina-Díaz IM, Robledo-Marenco ML, Velázquez-Fernández JB, Girón-Pérez MI, Ortega-Cervantes L, Maldonado-Vázquez WA, Rojas-García AE. Acetylcholinesterase and metallothionein in oysters (*Crassostrea corteziensis*) from a subtropical Mexican Pacific estuary. Ecotoxicology. 2010;19(4):819–25.
33. Géret F, Jouan A, Turpin V, Bebianno MJ, Cosson RP. Influence of metal exposure on metallothionein synthesis and lipid peroxidation in two bivalve mollusks:: the oyster (*Crassostrea gigas*) and the mussel (*Mytilus edulis*). Aquat Living Resour. 2002;15(1):61–6.
34. Gao JL, Ishizaki S, Nagashima Y. Purification and characterization of metal-binding proteins from the digestive gland of the Japanese scallop Mizuhopecten yessoensis. Fish Sci. 2016;82(2):337–45.

Chapter 3
Digestion and Absorption of Marine Shellfish Protein

Ming Du, Shaoyun Wang, Di Wu, Minbo Li, and Ximing Yang

Abstract Marine shellfish are rich in diverse bioactive components, with proteins, small peptides, and amino acids being particularly prominent. These components play a crucial role in the synthesis of hormones and enzymes in the human body, contributing to various physiological functions and offering significant health benefits. Marine shellfish proteins and their bioactive peptides hold broad application potential in the food, dietary supplement, and pharmaceutical industries, especially when processed using technologies like enzymatic engineering and fermentation. However, domestic research and industry still face challenges in maximizing protein utilization, particularly in achieving high-efficiency enzymatic hydrolysis. Protein digestion in the human body depends on a range of enzymes, primarily pepsin in the stomach and pancreatic enzymes in the small intestine. These enzymes break proteins down into smaller peptides, enabling their absorption and utilization by the body. This chapter further explores the digestion process of marine shellfish proteins, their bioactive properties, and their potential contributions to human health.

Keywords Shellfish proteins · Bioactivity · Absorption · Enzymes · Peptides · Nutrition

Aquatic proteins are not only exceptionally nutritious but also easily digestible and absorbable by the human body. Marine shellfish, in particular, are rich in proteins, peptides, amino acids, and other bioactive components. The nutritional benefits of protein-derived peptides primarily stem from proteins, peptides, and L-amino acids, with small peptides playing a more active role in biological processes than free

M. Du (✉)
College of Food Science and Engineering, Dalian Ocean University, Dalian, China

S. Wang
Biological Science and Engineering, Fuzhou University, Fuzhou, China

D. Wu · M. Li · X. Yang
Food Science and Engineering, Dalian Polytechnic University, Dalian, China

M. Du, S. Cheng (eds.), *Bioactive Proteins and Peptides from Marine Shellfish*,
https://doi.org/10.1007/978-981-95-3937-6_3

amino acids alone. As an effective source of protein supplementation, dietary proteins allow the human body to acquire small peptides and L-amino acids, which support the synthesis of hormones, enzymes, and structural proteins. Dietary proteins are also a major source of bioactive peptides. Some exist naturally in food, while others are produced through protease-catalyzed enzymatic hydrolysis. Modern bioengineering techniques, such as fermentation engineering and enzyme engineering, are increasingly used to develop marine shellfish protein resources. These approaches focus on high-value, resource-efficient, and eco-friendly utilization, making them an important means for the comprehensive exploitation of shellfish resources both domestically and internationally. Their applications span seasonings, health foods, nutritional products, and pharmaceuticals [1]. Currently, China faces certain bottlenecks in the enzymatic utilization of marine shellfish proteins, including an overabundance of repetitive low-level studies and a relative lack of advanced, in-depth enzymatic technologies. Thus, breaking through traditional enzymatic hydrolysis methods to enable high-value, eco-friendly development of marine shellfish protein resources has become a key research focus for the comprehensive utilization of shellfish resources in China [1].

Proteases hydrolyze proteins into peptides and amino acids, enhancing the solubility, emulsification, foaming capacity, viscosity, and flavor of proteins. This enzymatic process avoids amino acid degradation caused by acid or alkali hydrolysis, thereby preserving the nutritional value of proteins [2]. Protein digestion in the human body occurs under mild enzymatic conditions, a process with significant market potential. Additionally, enzymatic biotransformation markedly alters the structural properties of proteins. The human digestive tract is primarily composed of enzymes, water, inorganic substances, and mucus, with each component playing a distinct role in protein digestion and absorption. Key enzymes involved include salivary amylase, pepsin, trypsin, pancreatic lipase, chymotrypsin, sucrase, and maltase [3]. In mammals, serine proteases are critical for protein digestion. These enzymes are activated by conformational changes at their active sites, which involve specific amino acid residues, serine being a consistent component. Pepsin, chymotrypsin, and trypsin all belong to the serine protease family. Specifically, pepsin cleaves peptide bonds adjacent to aromatic amino acids or leucine residues at either the amino or carboxyl terminus. Chymotrypsin primarily targets hydrophobic amino acids at the carboxyl terminus of peptides. And trypsin, an endopeptidase, cleaves peptide bonds at the carboxyl terminus of arginine or lysine residues. Through enzymatic hydrolysis in the digestive tract, proteins are broken down to release bioactive peptide fragments. These fragments permeate the intestinal epithelium, enter the bloodstream, and reach various organs, tissues, and cells to exert their specific biological functions [1, 3]. Thus, studying the digestive and absorptive properties of marine shellfish proteins is of great significance.

3.1 Digestive Characteristics

3.1.1 Oyster

Oysters, belonging to the class Bivalvia, are primarily distributed in tropical and subtropical waters and are widely found along China's coastal areas. China boasts a rich diversity of oyster species, with major types including the Pacific oyster (*Crassostrea gigas*), Mexican oyster, Kumamoto oyster, and Hong Kong oyster. According to the 2024 Fishery Statistical Yearbook, China's marine aquaculture output of oysters reached 6.671 million tons in 2023, showing a sustained growth trend. Among these, the Pacific oyster stands out due to its superior breed, extensive cultivation scale, and highest production volume. Years of breeding efforts have yielded domesticated Pacific oysters with larger individuals, higher shells, and thicker meat, which exhibit significant growth advantages over various wild species. Renowned for their exceptional nutritional and medicinal value, oysters are regarded as a premium marine resource. They are high in protein, low in fat, and rich in various vitamins and minerals, making them an excellent nutritional source [4]. Oyster proteins are particularly abundant, accounting for approximately 7% of wet weight and up to 47.3% of dry weight. Additionally, oysters contain a variety of bioactive compounds, such as bioactive peptides, polysaccharides, taurine, eicosapentaenoic acid (EPA), and docosahexaenoic acid (DHA) [5]. The protein potential of oysters has attracted significant interest from nutritionists, clinicians, and medical researchers, and they are widely used as raw materials in conventional foods, health foods, and pharmaceuticals [4, 6, 7].

Pacific oysters (*Crassostrea gigas*), a species with a fully sequenced genome, are valued for their high production and protein content. Hydrolyzing their proteins *via* protease treatment or biological fermentation, followed by molecular weight-based peptide fractionation, has revealed multiple bioactive properties. Thus, the Pacific oyster stands as a high-quality protein source with broad developmental potential. However, common enzymatic hydrolysis methods face limitations regarding the in vivo bioactivity of the resulting peptides. When peptides produced by nonhuman digestive enzymes enter the human body, they may undergo secondary or repeated hydrolysis by gastrointestinal proteases, potentially impairing their original bioactivity [8]. Many peptides exhibit significantly reduced bioactivity in vivo compared to in vitro assays. In contrast, peptides hydrolyzed by homologous digestive proteases in the gastrointestinal tract can retain their original structure, minimizing further breakdown and avoiding bioactivity loss caused by gastrointestinal enzymes. During simulated gastric digestion, pepsin, a single protease, primarily cleaves residues like Phe-, Tyr-, and Leu-, breaking large protein molecules into longer peptide fragments and leading to relatively low hydrolysis rates in the gastric phase. By contrast, during the pancreatic digestion phase, pancreatic enzymes, a complex enzyme system, act synergistically to break down tissues into smaller monomers, releasing more protein content and enhancing trypsin activity [9, 10]. Trypsin primarily cleaves at Arg- and Lys- residues. In a study by Chen et al. on the simulated gastrointestinal digestion mechanism of Pacific oyster tissue, oyster proteins were continuously degraded into protein fragments or smaller peptides. The degree of hydrolysis (DH) of these proteins during digestion was measured using the trinitrobenzenesulfonic acid (TNBS) method (as shown in Fig. 3.1) [11]. After 1 h of pepsin digestion, the DH of Pacific oyster protein increased slightly from 12.78% to 16.86%. After adding pancreatic enzymes, DH rose to 23.3% within 1 h and peaked at 26.28% by the end of the 4-h digestion period. During simulated gastric digestion, pepsin's limited cleavage sites (targeting amino acids like Phe-, Tyr-, and Leu-) result in lower hydrolysis rates. In comparison, the combined action of pancreatic enzymes, thanks to their complex system, significantly enhances hydrolysis efficiency. Trypsin, which mainly cleaves at Arg- and Lys- residues, sees a slowing of hydrolysis rate increases after 2–4 h of digestion. This is likely because easily digestible proteins are already degraded in the early stages of enzyme activity, while more structurally stable proteins or longer peptides, due to disulfide bonds, are more resistant to further hydrolysis.

Based on Fig. 3.2, the molecular weight distribution of Pacific oyster protein during the simulated gastric digestion phase ranges from 10 to 200 kDa. The ~200 kDa band represents myosin, with bands at 160 kDa corresponding to myosin heavy chain and paramyosin, and a clear band around 41 kDa for actin, indicating ongoing release of proteins during pepsin digestion. After 1 h of pancreatin digestion, the 200 kDa band disappears, and multiple bands appear in the 14–200 kDa range, showing that myosin heavy chains have mostly broken down into smaller

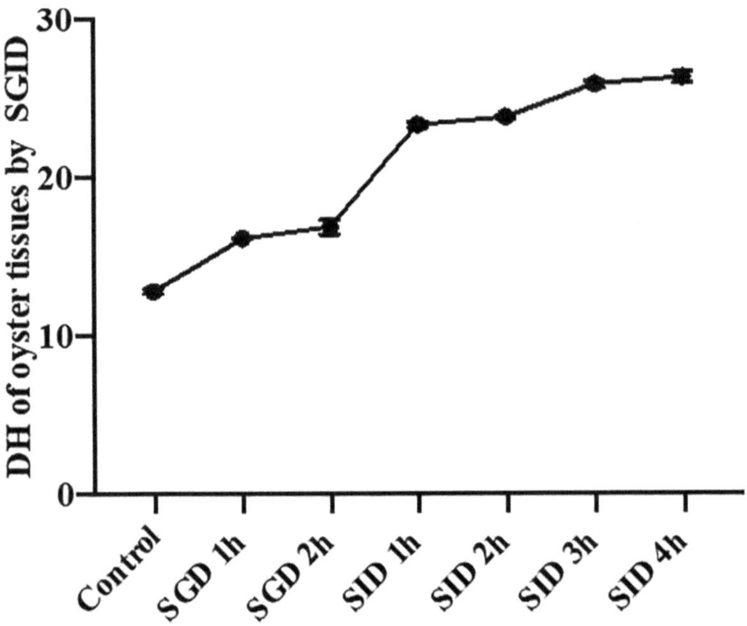

Fig. 3.1 Degree of hydrolysis of Pacific oyster protein during simulated gastrointestinal digestion

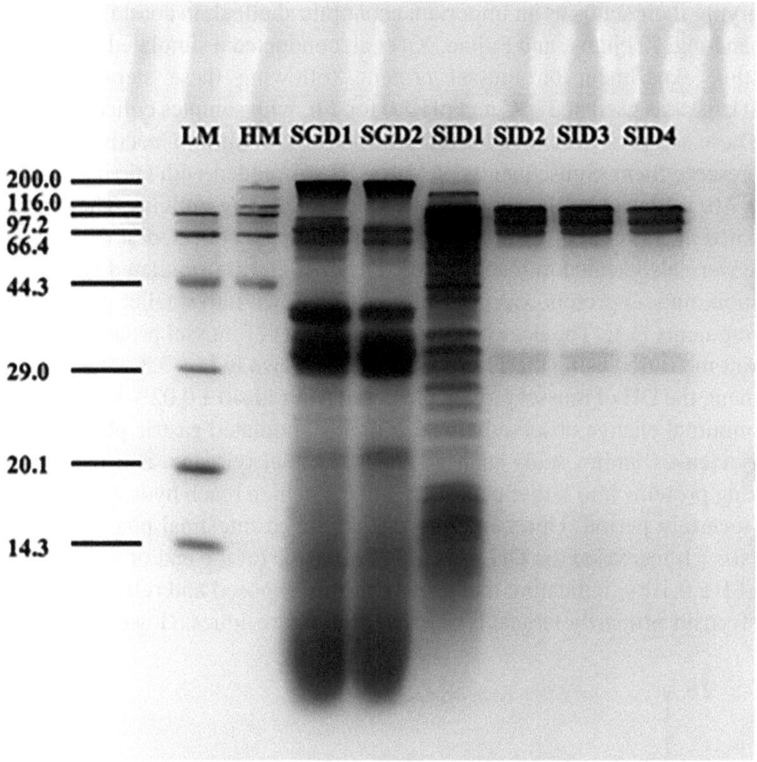

Fig. 3.2 SDS-PAGE protein electrophoresis analysis of supernatant from Pacific oyster during simulated gastrointestinal digestion

fragments, with soluble proteins further digested. After 2 h of pancreatin digestion, most bands vanish, the 30 kDa band becomes faint, and protein bands between 116 and 97 kDa remain distinct, gradually fading only after 4 h of digestion. In the early stage of pancreatin digestion, enzymatic activity is strong, rapidly degrading easily digestible proteins, while proteins or longer peptide structures that are stabilized by disulfide bonds remain relatively resistant. This result is consistent with the degree of hydrolysis observed in Pacific oyster protein during simulated gastrointestinal digestion.

3.1.2 *Mussel*

Mussels are bivalve marine mollusks belonging to the Mytilidae family (class Bivalvia), renowned for their high nutritional and medicinal value. In recent years, mussel production in China has continued to grow. According to the *2024 Fisheries Statistical Yearbook*, 2023 mussel aquaculture output reached 777,000 tons, solidifying their status as an important economic shellfish in coastal provinces such as Shandong, Zhejiang, and Fujian. Xu et al. conducted a simulated gastrointestinal digestion experiment on mussel protein, following these steps. First, pepsin (5000 U/g) was used at 37 °C and pH 2.0 for 2 h, with samples collected at 0, 1, and 2 h. These samples were then heated at 100 °C for 10 min to inactivate the enzyme and preserve them. Subsequently, 4 M NaOH was added with stirring to adjust the pH to 7.0, followed by the addition of trypsin (5000 U/g protein). The mixture was incubated at 37 °C and pH 8.0 for 3 h, with samples collected at 0, 1, 2, and 3 h. These were also heated to inactivate the enzyme. During simulated gastrointestinal digestion, mussel protein was gradually broken down into smaller protein and peptide fragments [12]. The degree of hydrolysis (DH) of mussel protein during digestion was measured using the TNBS method. As shown in Fig. 3.3, after 1 h of pepsin treatment, the DH of mussel protein increased from 11.46 ± 0.02% to 15.37 ± 0.04%, with minimal change observed after 2 h. In the simulated gastric phase, pepsin primarily cleaves amino acids such as phenylalanine, tyrosine, and leucine, mainly breaking proteins into larger peptide segments, which reach hydrolysis equilibrium after a certain period. Upon entering the simulated intestinal phase, trypsin treatment for 1 h increased the DH from 15.45 ± 0.07% (at the end of gastric digestion) to 16.61 ± 0.10%, indicating that trypsin further exposed and released protein content. Trypsin primarily targets lysine and arginine residues. However, little change

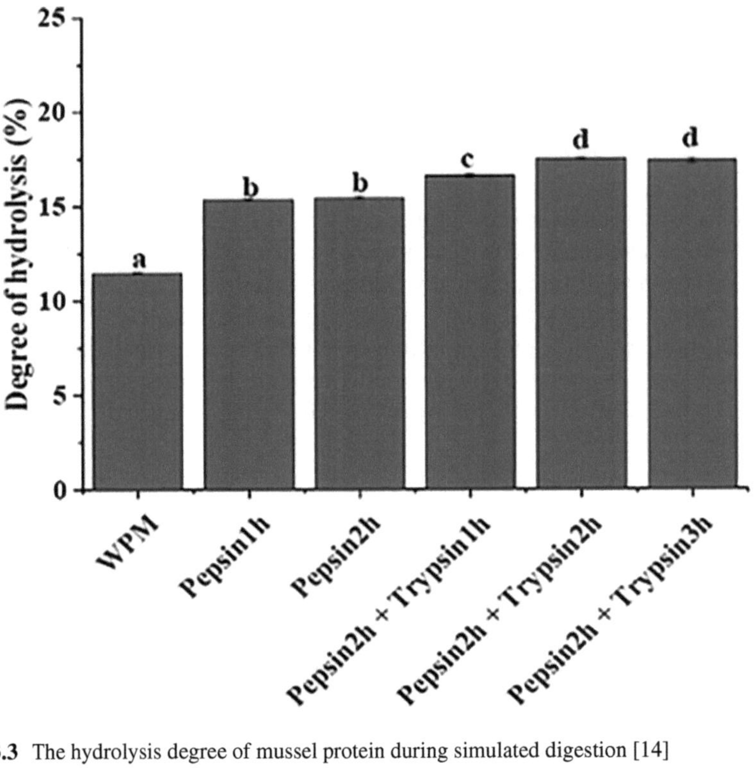

Fig. 3.3 The hydrolysis degree of mussel protein during simulated digestion [14]

in DH was observed after 2 and 3 h of trypsin digestion. This is likely because easily digestible protein fragments were fully degraded, while some fragments with disulfide bonds, having a more stable structure, were resistant to further hydrolysis or reached a stable peptide state [13].

The obtained samples were analyzed by SDS-PAGE to examine the protein composition. During the gastric digestion phase, pepsin mainly degraded large molecular weight proteins, and mussel protein was cleaved into fragments with molecular weights ranging from 37 to 250 kDa. Additionally, proteins or peptides with molecular weights between 10 and 37 kDa were released (Fig. 3.4) [14]. These hydrolyzed components (pepsin digestion for 1–2 h) completely disappeared during the intestinal digestion phase, indicating that the 10–37 kDa proteins or peptides were further degraded. In the trypsin digestion phase (1–3 h), these components were broken down into lower molecular weight bioactive peptides or free amino acids. This result is consistent with the analysis of the hydrolysis degree of mussel protein.

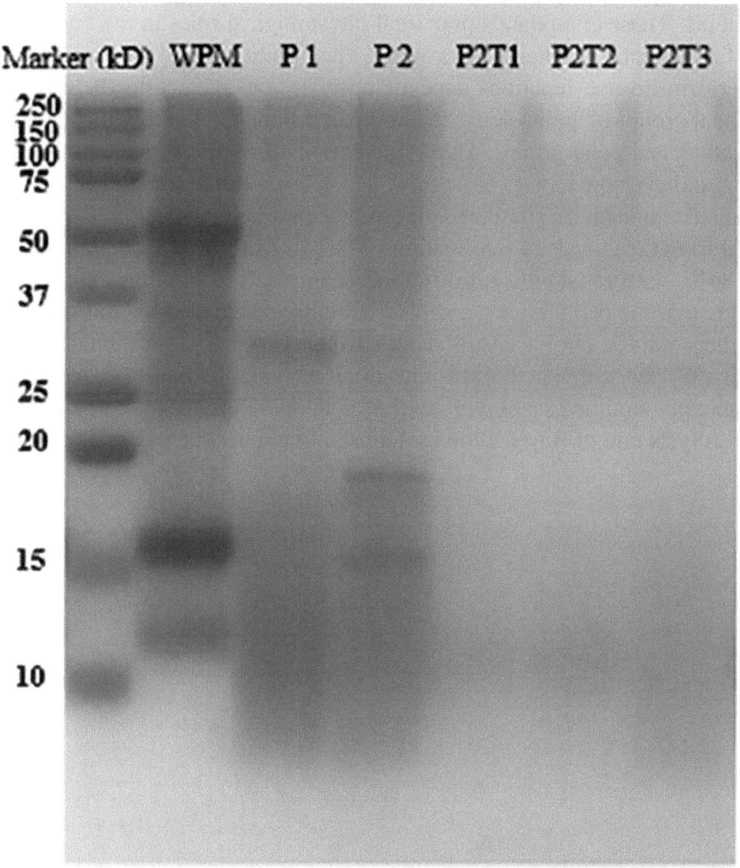

Fig. 3.4 SDS-PAGE of WPM after in vitro simulated gastric and intestinal digestion [14]

3.1.3 Scallop

The Bay scallop (*Chlamys farreri*), commonly known as dry scallop (derived from its adductor muscle) or sea fan, belongs to the Mollusca phylum, Bivalvia class, Pteriomorphia order, Pectinidae family, and the genus *Chlamys*. According to the *2024 Fisheries Statistical Yearbook*, total shellfish production from aquaculture and capture reached 16.46 million tons in 2023, accounting for 24% of relevant aquatic output. Bay scallops are rich in high-quality animal proteins and easily absorbable amino acids. Since scallop products primarily use the adductor muscle (i.e., the scallop column) as the main ingredient, domestic research on Bay scallops has focused largely on aquaculture, breeding, and heavy metal detection. While some studies have explored their application in seasoning development, research remains limited in areas such as deep processing, high-value product development, and the separation, purification, and functional analysis of their proteins or peptides [14–16].

Peptides and proteins are compounds formed by α-amino acids linked *via* peptide bonds. Typically, peptides containing more than 50 amino acids are classified as proteins. These compounds play vital physiological roles in the body and serve as the fundamental building blocks of life. Their ability to fold in an ordered manner and perform diverse functions depends critically on interactions between various functional groups of amino acids, including hydrophobic, hydrophilic, neutral, electronegative, and polar groups. These interactions drive the formation of secondary, tertiary, and even quaternary structures.

Jin et al. conducted a simulated digestion experiment on peptide-Ca^{2+} complexes derived from the gonads of Ezo scallops. The results showed a calcium dialysis rate of 41.86%, with no significant difference compared to pre-digestion levels. This confirms that the peptide-Ca^{2+} complex is highly stable, as Ca^{2+} did not dissociate from the complex during gastrointestinal digestion [17]. Additionally, Wu et al. investigated the simulated gastrointestinal enzymatic digestion mechanism of mechanically modified scallop protein. As shown in Fig. 3.5, after pepsin digestion, the hydrolysis rate of Bay scallop protein stabilized between 45 and 60 min. When

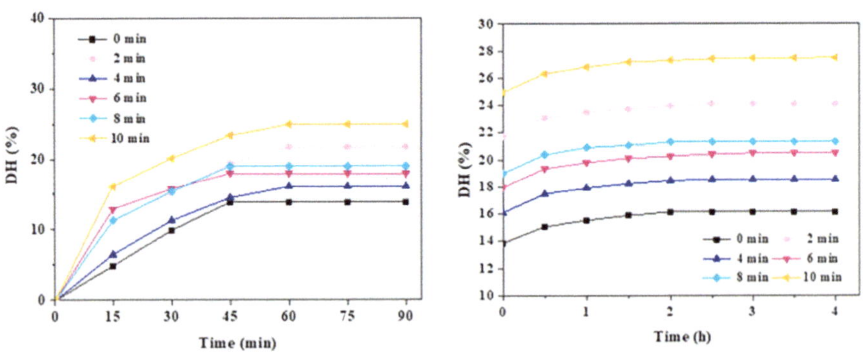

Fig. 3.5 Effect of simulated gastrointestinal digestion on the hydrolysis degree of *Chlamys farreri* protein [18]

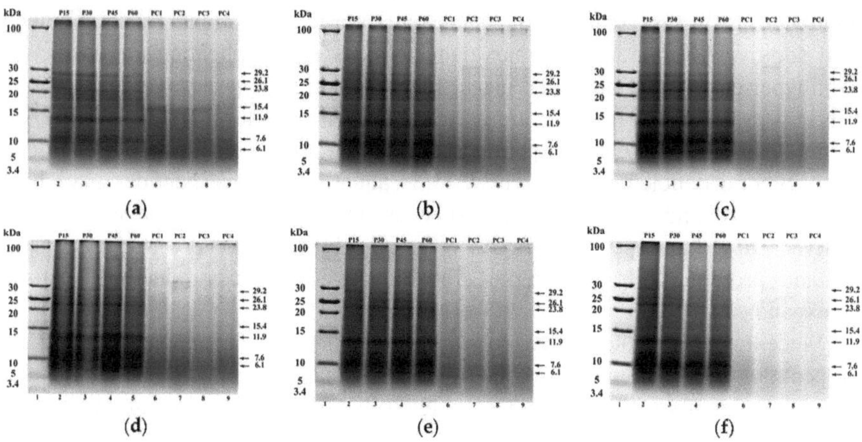

Fig. 3.6 Impact of simulated gastrointestinal digestion on the digestion characteristics of ball-milled *Chlamys farreri* protein [18]

the pH was subsequently adjusted to mimic the intestinal environment and trypsin was added, the hydrolysis rate increased rapidly in the first 60 min and reached complete hydrolysis within 3–4 h [18].

Figure 3.6 shows the Tricine-SDS-PAGE electrophoretic patterns of *Chlamys farreri* protein at different digestion time points after ball milling treatment. In the figure, P15, P30, P45, and P60 represent the protein digested for 15, 30, 45, and 60 min in the simulated gastric environment, respectively. PC1, PC2, PC3, and PC4 indicate the samples subjected to 1, 2, 3, and 4 h of trypsin hydrolysis after 60 min of gastric digestion [18]. The analysis results show that after 60 min of simulated gastric digestion, seven protein bands with molecular weights of 29.2, 26.1, 23.8, 15.4, 11.9, 7.6, and 6.1 kDa are clearly visible on the electrophoretic gel. Notably, the protein bands at 7.6 and 6.1 kDa gradually darken as the ball milling time increases. After 1 h of simulated intestinal digestion, proteins of 29.2, 26.1, and 23.8 kDa undergo significant hydrolysis, generating lower molecular weight proteins. With the increase in ball milling treatment time, the trypsin hydrolysis process becomes more thorough [19].

3.2 Absorption Characteristics

Bioactive peptides derived from aquatic proteins remain soluble and electrically neutral during intestinal digestion. They require low energy for transport, exhibit fast transport rates, and are less likely to saturate transporters. These peptides offer significant physiological functions, high safety, and diverse raw material sources, including low-value fish, shrimp, mollusks, algae, and their processing byproducts. Their bioactivities have been validated in cell and animal models, making them highly promising as dietary supplements, particularly in functional food ingredients and additives. For example, antioxidant peptides find applications in cosmetics. Antihypertensive peptides can replace side effect-prone hypertension medications. Anticancer/antitumor peptides are used for cancer prevention and treatment. And mineral absorption-promoting peptides serve as dietary supplements for individuals with mineral deficiencies. Currently, some aquatic bioactive peptides have been industrialized and commercialized, such as antihypertensive peptide beverages derived from Japanese sardines. As research advances, the prospects for using aquatic proteins as raw materials for bioactive peptide production continue to expand.

Since the 1970s, studies have found that some small-molecular-weight proteins or peptides can be directly absorbed by the intestinal mucosa without being hydrolyzed into amino acids. Subsequent research has shown that protein and peptide drugs can also be absorbed through mucosal routes, including the nasal cavity, oral cavity, and rectum. Intact peptides and proteins can cross the gastrointestinal wall into lymphatic vessels, entering the lymphatic system through two pathways (lymphatic and nonlymphatic tissue absorption). Amino acid absorption primarily relies on three types of transporters in small intestinal mucosal cells, which specialize in transporting neutral, acidic, and basic amino acids. During transport, amino acids bind to their specific transporters, traverse the mucosal cells, then dissociate to enter the cells, after which the transporters return to the mucosal surface for subsequent transport cycles. These binding and dissociation processes are catalyzed by specific enzymes and require energy, primarily supplied by adenosine triphosphate (ATP).

3.2.1 Absorption Mechanisms

Traditional protein nutrition theory posits that once ingested proteins are first degraded by endopeptidases in the digestive tract into smaller oligopeptides, which are then broken down by exopeptidases into free amino acids for absorption [20]. In the 1960s, Newey et al. were the first to propose that small peptides could be absorbed intact, a theory later confirmed by Hara et al., who identified peptide transporters on intestinal mucosal cells, providing evidence that small peptides can enter the bloodstream directly through these cells [21]. Today, protein absorption theory has evolved into a comprehensive model. After limited digestion in the stomach, proteins enter the small intestine, where they are further broken down by pancreatic and intestinal enzymes into free amino acids and small peptides. These small peptides are then hydrolyzed in the intestinal mucosa into amino acids, dipeptides, and tripeptides for absorption, with larger peptides also being absorbed intact. Amino acid and peptide absorption occur *via* distinct pathways. Free amino acids are actively transported through four systems (specializing in neutral, basic, acidic amino acids, and imino acids), while peptide absorption is independent of concentration gradients.

Before being fully absorbed in the small intestine, peptides encounter multiple physical barriers, including the unstirred water layer, mucus layer, intestinal epithelial cells, and tight junctions. The composition of the intestinal barrier determines its permeability, and the unstirred water layer, located on the surface of intestinal epithelial cells, serves as the first physical barrier for intact peptide transport. This 100–800 nm thick layer plays a critical role in peptide transport. Notably, hydrophobic peptides must form micelles to traverse it [22]. As intestinal viscosity increases and chyme mixing weakens, the unstirred water layer thickens, slowing the transfer rate to absorption sites and impeding peptide absorption. Covering the tips and spaces between intestinal villi, this layer exhibits high viscoelasticity and adhesiveness, with a structure similar to a hydrogel. It contains highly branched polysaccharides and negatively charged mucins [23]. The average thickness of the intestinal mucus layer in humans is approximately 0.2 μm, functioning as a selective membrane that allows nutrient passage while blocking most bacteria and pathogens. As bioactive peptides traverse this layer, their diffusion is hindered by chemical interactions (e.g., hydrogen bonding, electrostatic and hydrophobic interactions) and physical entanglements with mucus polymers. This slowed diffusion reduces peptide access to epithelial cells, impacting absorption rates, particularly for hydrophobic peptides, whose transport and absorption time within the mucus layer is significantly influenced by the layer's rheological and physicochemical properties. In contrast, hydrophilic peptides are largely unaffected by the mucus layer [24].

After traversing the mucus layer, peptides must cross either intestinal epithelial cells or tight junctions to reach the bloodstream, where they can exert their physiological functions. Intestinal epithelial cells form a monolayer lining the intestinal lumen, regulating substance transport from the apical to the basal layer. These cells comprise enterocytes (which absorb nutrients), goblet cells (which secrete mucus), and immune-responsive cells [25]. Despite being a single-cell layer spanning approximately 400 m^2 in the human intestine, this epithelial layer serves as a significant physical barrier. Given the lipophilic nature of epithelial cells, hydrophilic peptides have limited capacity for transmembrane transport [26]. Additionally, as peptides move between adjacent epithelial cells, they encounter tight junctions, a key permeability barrier that limits the paracellular flow of water, ions, and solutes, thereby reducing permeability for large peptides [26]. Tight junction permeability varies among different animal cells, and epithelial cells can transiently modify these junctions to allow larger solutes to pass through. Connected to the cytoskeleton, tight junctions and epithelial cells form a dynamic barrier system, where permeability governs the overall barrier function of the intestinal epithelium.

3.2.2 Methods of Peptide Absorption Efficiency Measuring

The Caco-2 cell line is widely used as a model for studying intestinal barrier functions. Originally derived from human colon adenocarcinoma cells, Caco-2 cells spontaneously differentiate during culture to form a monolayer that exhibits various morphological and functional characteristics of small intestinal cells. For example, Chen et al. used this model to examine the peptide absorption and transport of hydrolysates from simulated gastrointestinal digestion of *Crassostrea gigas* in Caco-2 cells. Figure 3.7 illustrates that after adding 500 μg/mL of peptide to the apical side (AP) of Caco-2 cells, samples were collected from both the AP and basolateral (BL) sides at 15, 30, 60, and 120 min. The peptides in the medium were then quantitatively measured using liquid chromatography-mass spectrometry (LC-MS). After 15 min of incubation, the peptide concentration on the AP side was 322.99 ± 153.54 μg/mL, while the BL side concentration was 5.80 ± 0.50 μg/mL. At 30 min, the peptide concentration on the AP side dropped to 252.28 ± 89.54 μg/mL, with no significant change in the BL side concentration. By 120 min, the AP side concentration further decreased to 193.19 ± 11.47 μg/mL, while the BL side concentration rose to 6.77 ± 0.47 μg/mL. This data indicates an absorption efficiency of approximately 1% for the peptide P-CG-01 across intestinal cells in vitro. Additionally, when the concentrations from the AP and BL sides were converted to total mass per unit volume, the combined mass was lower than the initial concentration in the peptide stock solution. This discrepancy may be attributed to degradation of peptides by proteases, such as carboxypeptidases, aminopeptidases, and endopeptidases, secreted by the brush border epithelium on the intestinal cells.

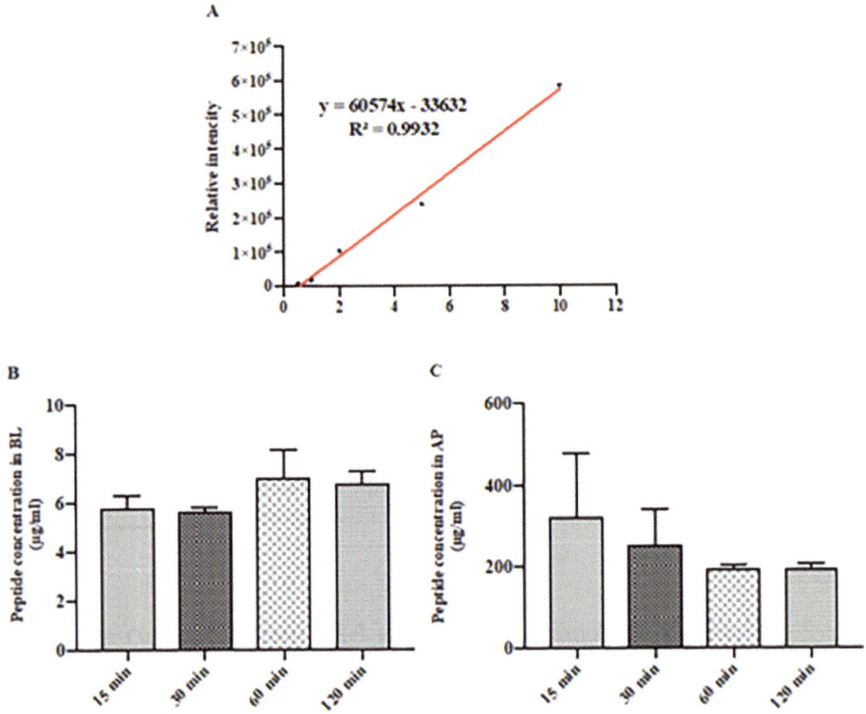

Fig. 3.7 Absorption of *Crassostrea gigas* peptides by Caco-2 cells. (a) Standard curve of P-CG-01 detected by LC-MS; (b) P-CG-01 concentration in the BL compartment; (c) P-CG-01 concentration in the AP compartment [27]

In mammals, the absorption rate of amino acid residues in small peptides is generally faster than that of free amino acids. This is because small peptides are less susceptible to further hydrolysis in the intestine, enabling more complete absorption into the bloodstream. Once in circulation, these small peptides can directly contribute to tissue protein synthesis. Additionally, organs and tissues such as the liver, kidneys, and skin can effectively utilize small peptides. Studies have demonstrated that compared to free amino acids, small peptides are more readily absorbed and utilized by the body and are less affected by antinutritional factors.

Chen et al. conducted a gavage experiment in mice to examine peptide absorption. After administering the peptides, blood samples were collected from the orbital sinus at intervals of 10, 20, 30 min, 1, 2, 4, 6, and 12 h to measure serum peptide concentration. As shown in Fig. 3.8, peptides were detectable in serum as early as 10 min post-gavage, rapidly reaching an initial concentration peak. This result aligns with in vitro absorption findings, indicating a high absorption efficiency, likely due to the peptide's favorable water solubility. At this point, the serum peptide concentration was 2.36 ± 0.71 μg/mL. After 2 h, a second peak was observed at approximately 1.54 ± 0.71 μg/mL. The peptides remained detectable in the bloodstream for up to 4 h, and by 6 h, the concentration had nearly disappeared, with no detectable peptides after 12 h. These findings indicate that the peptide can rapidly enter the bloodstream, be effectively absorbed, and remain in circulation for approximately 4 h [11].

Studies have shown that the primary form in which the human body absorbs protein is peptides. The absorption mechanism exhibits several key characteristics. First, peptides travel directly from the mouth and stomach to the small intestine,

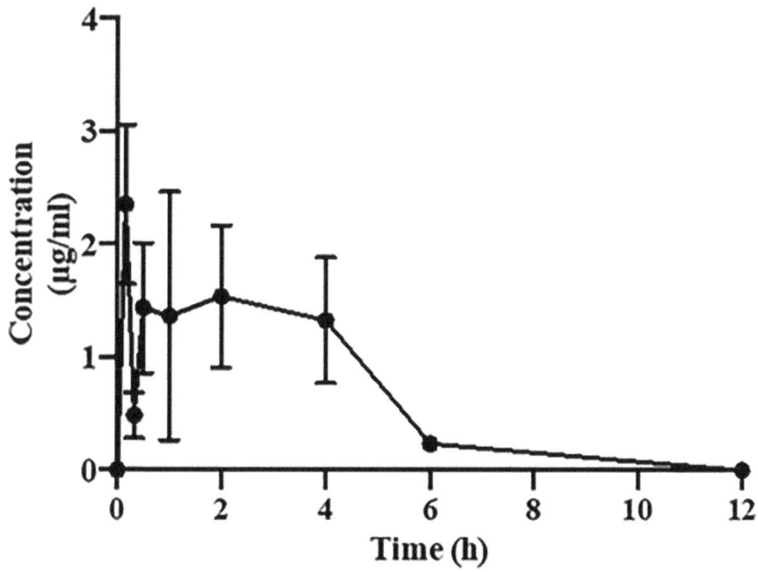

Fig. 3.8 Peptide content in mouse serum [27]

where they are absorbed before entering the bloodstream, organs, and cellular tissues to promptly exert physiological and biological functions. Second, this absorption process is unaffected by endogenous proteolytic enzymes, pancreatic enzymes, or amylase. It also avoids interference from digestive enzymes like pepsin, as well as acidic and alkaline substances in the digestive system, factors that might otherwise cause damage or secondary hydrolysis. Additionally, small peptides protect amino acids during absorption, preventing their degradation. Importantly, peptides can chelate with calcium and zinc ions, enhancing the absorption of these trace elements and facilitating their transport to cells, organs, and tissues throughout the body. Finally, peptides act as messengers in the body, transmitting information as neurotransmitters to ensure coordinated functioning of various systems, organs, and tissues. While considerable progress has been made in developing functional foods from aquatic proteins, most studies remain at the experimental stage. Before these functional products can enter commercial production, further research is needed on their bioavailability, compatibility with different food matrices, long-term stability, and in vivo efficacy.

3.3 Summary

Protein intake from a normal diet provides the body with various small peptides and L-amino acids, which are used to synthesize hormones, enzymes, and proteins. Marine shellfish proteins, in particular, are more easily digested and absorbed by the human body due to their high nutritional value. Enzymatic hydrolysis catalyzed by proteases is a primary source of bioactive peptides. After being hydrolyzed by digestive enzymes, proteins release specific bioactive peptide fragments that can cross the intestinal epithelium, enter the bloodstream, and reach organs, tissues, and cells to exert their functional properties. Thus, advancing and optimizing traditional enzymatic hydrolysis techniques to achieve high-value and environmentally sustainable development of marine shellfish protein resources is of significant research importance, especially regarding the digestive and absorptive properties of marine shellfish and their related applications.

References

1. Wu G, Fanzo J, Miller DD, Pingali P, Post M, Steiner JL, Thalacker-Mercer AE. Production and supply of high-quality food protein for human consumption: sustainability, challenges, and innovations. Ann N Y Acad Sci. 2014;1321(1):1–19.
2. Shankar R, Upadhyay PK, Kumar M. Protease enzymes: highlights on potential of proteases as therapeutics agents. Int J Pept Res Ther. 2021;27(2):1281–96.
3. Dyer RP, Weiss GA. Making the cut with protease engineering. Cell Chem Biol. 2022;29(2):177–90.

4. Levine H, Remington RE, Culp FB, Anderson CB. The value of the oyster in nutritional anemia. J Nutr. 1931;4(4):469–81.
5. Cong X, Wang Q, Sun C, Yu F, Chen L, Sun Z, Shi H, Xue C, Li Z. Temperature effects on the nutritional quality in Pacific oysters during ultraviolet depuration. J Sci Food Agric. 2022;102(4):1651–9.
6. Ulagesan S, Krishnan S, Nam T-J, Choi Y-H. A review of bioactive compounds in oyster shell and tissues. Front Bioeng Biotechnol. 2022;10:913839.
7. Adzigbli L, Hao R, Jiao Y, Deng Y, Du X, Wang Q, Huang R. Immune response of pearl oysters to stress and diseases. Rev Aquac. 2020;12(2):513–23.
8. Yang M, Su S, Cheng S, Wang Z, Du M. Absorption and transport properties of a codfish-derived peptide and its protective effect on bone loss in ovariectomized mice. Food Funct. 2024;15(7):3496–506.
9. Wang X, Yu H, Xing R, Liu S, Chen X, Li P. Optimization of oyster (*Crassostrea talienwhanensis*) protein hydrolysates using response surface methodology. Molecules. 2020;25(12):2844.
10. Chen T, Zhang F, Chen S, Zhao Y, Huang X, Huang F, Li C. Improvement mechanism of umami peptides in oyster juice by cooperative enzymolysis of alcalase and trypsin based on peptidomics and molecular docking. J Food Compos Anal. 2024;132:106326.
11. Chen H, Cheng S, Fan F, Tu M, Xu Z, Du M. Identification and molecular mechanism of antithrombotic peptides from oyster proteins released in simulated gastro-intestinal digestion. Food Funct. 2019;10(9):5426–35.
12. Xu Z, Chen H, Fan F, Shi P, Tu M, Cheng S, Wang Z, Du M. Bone formation activity of an osteogenic dodecapeptide from blue mussels (*Mytilus edulis*). Food Funct. 2019;10(9):5616–25.
13. Chen H, Xu Z, Fan F, Shi P, Tu M, Wang Z, Du M. Identification and mechanism evaluation of a novel osteogenesis promoting peptide from Tubulin alpha-1C chain in *Crassostrea gigas*. Food Chem. 2019;272:751–7.
14. Xu Z, Zhao F, Chen H, Xu S, Fan F, Shi P, Tu M, Wang Z, Du M. Nutritional properties and osteogenic activity of enzymatic hydrolysates of proteins from the blue mussel (*Mytilus edulis*). Food Funct. 2019;10(12):7745–54.
15. Song L, Wang L, Zhang H, Wang M. The immune system and its modulation mechanism in scallop. Fish Shellfish Immunol. 2015;46(1):65–78.
16. Beltrán-Lugo AI, Maeda-Martínez AN, Pacheco-Aguilar R, Nolasco-Soria HG. Seasonal variations in chemical, physical, textural, and microstructural properties of adductor muscles of Pacific lions-paw scallop (*Nodipecten subnodosus*). Aquaculture. 2006;258(1):619–32.
17. Jin WG, Du YN, Pei JJ, Zhao J, Tang Y, Shang WH, Wu HT, Zhu BW. Characterization and antioxidant activity of Maillard reaction products from a scallop (*Patinopecten yessoensis*) gonad hydrolysates-sugar model system. J Food Meas Charact. 2018;12(4):2883–91.
18. Wu D, Wu C, Chen H, Wang Z, Yu C, Du M. Effect of ball mill treatment on the physicochemical properties and digestibility of protein extracts generated from scallops (*Chlamys farreri*). Int J Mol Sci. 2018;19(531):1–12.
19. Wu D, Wu C, Tu M, Yu C, Du M. Identification and analysis of bioactive peptides from scallops (*Chlamys farreri*) protein by simulated gastrointestinal digestion. J Food Process Preserv. 2018;42(9):e13760.
20. Newey H, Sanford PA, Smyth DH. Uranyl ions and intestinal hexose transfer. Nature. 1965;205(4969):389–90.
21. Nishiyama Y, Planque S, Hara M, Watanabe K, Xu X, Taguchi H, Sigurdsson EM, O'Nuallain B, Murray I, Friedland RP, Fukuchi K-I, Massey R, Paul S. P4-201: beneficial catalytic autoimmunity to beta-amyloid peptide. Alzheimers Dement. 2012;8(4S_Part_19):P706.
22. Paone P, Cani PD. Mucus barrier, mucins and gut microbiota: the expected slimy partners. Gut. 2020;69(12):2232–43.
23. Johansson MEV, Hansson GC. Immunological aspects of intestinal mucus and mucins. Nat Rev Immunol. 2016;16(10):639–49.

24. Johansson MEV, Larsson JMH, Hansson GC. The two mucus layers of colon are organized by the MUC2 mucin, whereas the outer layer is a legislator of host–microbial interactions. Proc Natl Acad Sci USA. 2011;108(supplement_1):4659–65.
25. Pelaseyed T, Hansson GC. Membrane mucins of the intestine at a glance. J Cell Sci. 2020;133(5):jcs240929.
26. Ermund A, Schütte A, Johansson MEV, Gustafsson JK, Hansson GC. Studies of mucus in mouse stomach, small intestine, and colon. I. Gastrointestinal mucus layers have different properties depending on location as well as over the Peyer's patches. Am J Physiol Gastrointest Liver Physiol. 2013;305(5):G341–7.
27. Chen H, Shi P, Xu Z, Fan F, Wang Z, Du M. Oral administration of oyster peptide prevents bone loss in ovariectomized mice. eFood. 2020;1(4):298–309.

Chapter 4
Preparation and Identification of Marine Shellfish Peptides

Ming Du, Hui Chen, Shuzhen Cheng, Geng Cao, and Jun Feng

Abstract In recent years, consumers have become much more aware of how diet connects to health. People are increasingly recognizing that functional foods can benefit health when combined with a balanced lifestyle. This growing awareness has boosted demand for foods that support well-being, help people live longer, and reduce disease risk. Enzymatic hydrolysis offers an effective way to use shellfish proteins in many functional food products. This technique often uses methods like membrane filtration or fractionation to refine protein extracts. Bioactive peptides from shellfish proteins do more than supply essential nutrients. They also provide various health benefits. To understand the biological activities of these peptides, researchers need to analyze their specific sequences in detail. This chapter will focus on the processes used to extract, hydrolyze, separate, and identify shellfish proteins. Additionally, it will explore how bioinformatics and molecular simulation can predict the functional properties of shellfish protein peptides.

Keywords Marine shellfish · Protein · Peptides · Identification · Preparation

M. Du (✉)
College of Food Science and Engineering, Dalian Ocean University, Dalian, China

H. Chen
Food Science and Engineering, Zhejiang University of Technology, Zhejiang, China

S. Cheng
School of Food Science and Technology, Dalian Polytechnic University, Dalian, China

G. Cao · J. Feng
Food Science and Engineering, Dalian Polytechnic University, Dalian, China

M. Du, S. Cheng (eds.), *Bioactive Proteins and Peptides from Marine Shellfish*,
https://doi.org/10.1007/978-981-95-3937-6_4

4.1 Protein Extraction and Preparation

4.1.1 Classification and Properties

Muscle proteins are classified into three groups based on their solubility characteristics: water-soluble, salt-soluble, and insoluble proteins. These proteins were extracted using a phosphate buffer solution, which effectively isolates each protein type while minimizing impact on their native properties. Water-soluble proteins are a general category encompassing various water-soluble (or dilute salt-soluble) proteins present in the sarcoplasm of muscle cells, including numerous metabolism-related enzyme proteins that primarily influence meat flavor and color. These proteins are characterized by low molecular weight, high solubility, and strong bioactivity, including diverse antioxidant properties. Salt-soluble proteins are vital components of muscle tissue, consisting of complexes such as myosin, actin, actomyosin, and regulatory proteins that play significant roles in meat's water-holding capacity, emulsifying properties, and gelation abilities. Finally, insoluble proteins—known as stromal proteins—include collagen and elastin, which remain as residues after the extraction of water- and salt-soluble proteins. As major components of connective tissue, stromal proteins affect meat tenderness and elasticity, with their proportion of total protein content varying notably across different shellfish species.

4.1.2 Extraction and Component Analysis

Traditional protein extraction methods include aqueous extraction, heat extraction, and acid/alkali dissolution combined with isoelectric precipitation. Selecting a suitable extraction method is crucial to reduce protein denaturation and prevent loss of functional properties. In shellfish protein extraction, precooled phosphate buffer is usually applied first. Subsequent steps involve blending, homogenization, extraction, centrifugation, precipitation, acetone washing, and solubilization, which together yield sarcoplasmic protein components. The resulting precipitate is then dispersed in cold phosphate buffer, followed by homogenization, extraction, stirring, and centrifugation. Through this process, a supernatant containing myofibrillar proteins is obtained, while the remaining precipitate comprises stromal proteins. Dialysis may be employed to further remove salts from the myofibrillar protein component [1]. In terms of protein content, oysters contain the highest proportion of water-soluble proteins at 38%, followed by salt-soluble proteins at 31% and insoluble proteins at 26%. In fish muscle, sarcoplasmic proteins typically account for approximately 20–50% of total protein content, while myofibrillar proteins make up 50–70%. For instance, tilapia has lower water-soluble protein levels than oysters but significantly higher salt-soluble protein levels, reaching 49%. Similarly, the protein content profiles of *Litopenaeus vannamei* and *Pinctada martensii* follow the same pattern observed in the comparison between tilapia and oysters. Specifically, tilapia, shrimp, and *Pinctada martensii* all contain less water-soluble protein than oysters, while their salt-soluble protein content is higher than that of oysters [2]. Commercial mussel protein powder, including 58% proteins and 23% polysaccharides, exhibits an extraction yield of almost 40% for alkali-soluble proteins, which represent 30.88% of the raw material, establishing it as the predominant protein fraction. Albumin comprises 6.3% of the raw material, whereas globulins and alcohol-soluble proteins are found in minimal quantities. Alkaline extraction followed by acid precipitation is generally performed at a solid-to-liquid ratio of 1:30, a pH of 11.5, and a temperature of 35 °C, with precipitation occurring at pH 3.5, yielding a mussel protein isolate of over 80% and a purity of 74%.

4.2 Enzymatic Preparation and Purification

4.2.1 Enzymatic Preparation of Peptides

The selection of shellfish materials for peptide production should be consistent with industrial-scale production requirements and of equivalent quality to proteins generated from other sources [3]. While there is no single standard for enzyme selection, various enzyme preparations are currently applied in the production of shellfish-derived peptides. Nonetheless, pinpointing the ideal enzyme to produce peptides with specific bioactivity continues to be a challenge. Table 4.1 summarizes commonly used enzymes for shellfish protein hydrolysis and their characteristics. Notably, while most proteases are endopeptidases, flavor protease is a blend of exopeptidases and endopeptidases, which can alleviate bitterness often encountered in extensively hydrolyzed peptides.

To maintain constant product quality per ISO standards, the hydrolysis reaction requires continuous monitoring. The degree of hydrolysis (DH), defined as the ratio of cleaved peptide bonds to total bonds, serves as the primary metric. While multiple analytical methods exist, the pH-stat technique remains the most extensively validated approach for DH determination [4]. The pH-stat technique regulates pH levels (above 6.5) by titrating the released α-amino groups using an alkali. The correlation between DH and alkali consumption is articulated as follows.

$$\mathrm{DH\%} = B \times \mathrm{Nb} \times \frac{1}{\alpha} \times \frac{1}{\mathrm{MP}} \times \frac{1}{h_{\mathrm{tot}}} \times 100$$

Table 4.1 Commonly used proteases and their enzymatic hydrolysis conditions

Enzymes	Optimum pH	Temperature (°C)	Time	Degree of hydrolysis (%DH)
Alkaline protease	6.5–8.5	60	30 min to 3 h	15–25
Flavor protease	5.0–7.0	50–55	10 min to 3 h	–
Neutral protease	5.5–7.5	45–55	30 min to 3 h	10–15
Compound protease	7–8	50	30 min to 3 h	10–20
Pepsin	1–2	37	1 to 2 h	10–15
Trypsin	7.8–8.5	37	1 to 4 h	10–20

In this formula, B represents the volume of alkali added (mL), Nb is the equivalent concentration of alkali (mM), α is the average dissociation degree of α-amino groups, MP denotes the grams of protein in the reaction mixture, and h_{tot} represents the total peptide bond content (meq/g). The pH-stat method's principles have been widely applied in kinetic studies, where the degree of hydrolysis (DH) serves as an indicator of enzyme hydrolysis efficiency.

When enzymatic hydrolysis is employed to create peptides with specific biological activity, maintaining batch-to-batch consistency of hydrolyzed peptide components is critical. Protein hydrolysates can be classified based on the molecular weight of the peptide fragments produced during hydrolysis. Size-exclusion chromatography (SEC) is frequently utilized as a quantitative supplement to DH measurements [5], particularly for fractionating and producing bioactive peptides in the 100–7000 Da range. This method typically employs gel-filled chromatography columns, with acetonitrile-water solutions as mobile phases, to achieve effective separation.

4.2.2 Peptides Purification

Bioactive peptide hydrolysates typically show high complexity, making it challenging to identify specific bioactive peptides. Effective separation techniques are therefore essential to reduce compositional complexity and isolate functionally relevant peptides [6]. Separating and purifying peptides is important for understanding how they work and what they are made of. To achieve effective separation, methods are selected based on properties like molecular weight, polarity, and isoelectric point. Common techniques include electrophoresis, reverse-phase high-performance liquid chromatography (RP-HPLC), gel filtration chromatography, ion exchange chromatography, affinity chromatography, and ultrafiltration. Each of these offers different advantages for different peptide characteristics.

1. Electrophoresis

Electrophoresis (EP) separates proteins and peptides by exploiting differences in their charge and molecular weight under an electric field. Polyacrylamide gel electrophoresis (SDS-PAGE) can separate proteins of different molecular weights, while two-dimensional electrophoresis (2-DE) effectively separates proteins based on isoelectric points and molecular weights in two dimensions. Additionally, various capillary electrophoresis methods (CE)—including capillary gel electrophoresis, capillary isoelectric focusing, capillary isotachophoresis, and capillary zone electrophoresis—are widely applied in protein and peptide purification. EP is known for its high separation efficiency, speed, resolution, and selectivity. Whether used alone or in combination with other methods, EP achieves reliable separation results, though it may sometimes lead to peptide activity loss.

2. Reversed-Phase High-Performance Liquid Chromatography

Reversed-phase high-performance liquid chromatography (RP-HPLC) is a popular technique for peptide separation. It works by hydrophobic interactions, in which nonpolar or weakly polar peptide molecules connect to the nonpolar stationary phase (octadecylsilane-bonded silica gel). This interaction weakens as the polarity of the mobile phase shifts, allowing solute molecules to be eluted and separated. RP-HPLC provides great resolution, sensitivity, and effective separation while remaining simple to use and capable of high-throughput automated analysis of target peptides. However, the equipment is expensive, and it may not be as effective in retaining small, hydrophilic peptides.

3. Size-Exclusion Chromatography

Size-exclusion chromatography (SEC) separates molecules depending on their molecular size as they travel through a gel having sieve-like characteristics. This separation technique permits components to elute at different rates due to varied migration pathways, making it ideal for studying peptide molecular weight distribution and fractionation. SEC enables effective separation, quick processing, and reduces the danger of product denaturation. However, it may not always attain the desired purity level on its alone; combining SEC with other purification procedures frequently yields peptides of higher purity or activity.

4. Ion Exchange Chromatography

Ion exchange chromatography (IEC) separates peptides by exploiting the electrostatic attraction of ions in the peptide sample (anions or cations) to oppositely charged groups on the stationary phase. By changing the ionic strength or pH of the elution buffer, IEC may separate peptides and proteins based on their charge characteristics, resulting in successful purification. IEC is carried out using either cation or anion exchange columns, depending on the target compounds. This method preserves peptide bioactivity and, when combined with SEC, often produces optimum separation results. However, finding adequate ion exchange columns and fine-tuning elution conditions can be difficult tasks.

5. Ultrafiltration

Ultrafiltration (UF) is a popular technology for separating tiny molecules that is simple to use and requires minimal equipment. Its primary idea is to exploit the pressure difference at both ends of the membrane to drive and hold proteins and peptides with molecular weights ranging from 1 to 500 kDa. Ultrafiltration can save materials, increase peptide purity, and keep peptides active; however, it is only suitable for initial separation and not for separating a specific type of peptide. The development of ultrafiltration technology should focus on the study and development of new membrane separation materials with high selectivity and stability, as well as new ultrafiltration techniques.

6. Affinity Chromatography

Affinity chromatography (AC) is a separation process that relies on the reversible specific binding of an immobilized ligand to the component to be separated. Affinity chromatography is classified into immunoaffinity chromatography, nucleic acid affinity chromatography, metal chelate affinity chromatography, and so on. The key advantages of affinity chromatography are its excellent specificity, high resolution, good adsorption impact on unstable active compounds, and reusability; nonetheless, it is mostly utilized for the purification of antibodies and glycoproteins and has a limited range of applications.

7. Phosphopeptide Purification

Multiple methods exist for the isolation or enrichment of phosphopeptides, all relying on differential interactions between phosphopeptides and metals, such as titanium dioxide [6]. Adenosine triphosphate (ATP) has been shown to function as a very sensitive and selective agent for phosphopeptide extraction. Likewise, glycopeptides have been isolated from intricate materials employing various methodologies. Hydrophilic interaction liquid chromatography (HILIC) for glycopeptide extraction employs diverse stationary phases, including microcrystalline cellulose and zwitterionic substances. Separation and extraction of glycopeptides are generally accomplished using chemical agents such as boronic acid and hydrazine.

4.3 Peptide Sequence Identification

Sequential separation and identification techniques, such as matrix-assisted laser desorption/ionization time-of-flight mass spectrometry (MALDI-QTOF-MS), ultra-performance liquid chromatography time-of-flight mass spectrometry (UPLC-QTOF-MS), and capillary electrophoresis tandem mass spectrometry (CE-QTOF-MS), can be employed to isolate highly bioactive components. Figure 4.1 illustrates the workflow for the preparation [7], purification, and identification of bioactive peptides. Precise identification is crucial as these peptide sequences have substantial ramifications for human health; subsequent to identification, peptides are synthesized for the assessment of in vitro biological activity. Innovative strategies that incorporate bioinformatics, mass spectrometry, multi-omics methodologies (including proteomics and peptidomics), and enzymatic assays enhance the accuracy of identifying functional peptides from target proteins, supported by advancements in genomics, proteomics, foodomics, and computational analysis.

As sample complexity escalates in proteomics, the identification of peptide sequences with analogous molecular weights becomes increasingly difficult. The resolution of the mass spectrometer substantially influences the accuracy of peptide assignment; nonetheless, precise mass alone frequently proves inadequate for recognizing peptide sequences. Consequently, peptide analysis depends on instruments proficient in tandem fragmentation to provide supplementary sequencing data. The predominant fragmentation method employed in peptidomics is collision-induced dissociation (CID). In conjunction with CID, electron transfer dissociation (ETD) and high-energy CID facilitate sequence analysis, each yielding unique yet complementary outcomes for a thorough peptide profile.

In database searching, tandem mass spectrometry data are aligned with theoretical spectra derived from protein databases to deduce peptide sequences. Conversely,

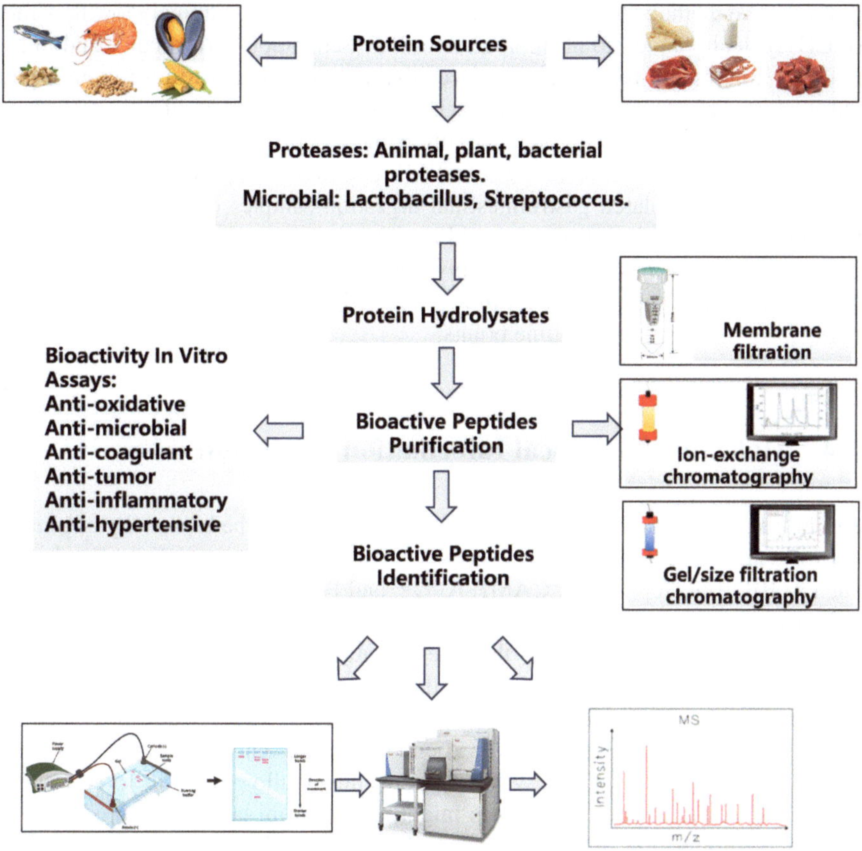

Fig. 4.1 Principle of preparation, purification, and identification of bioactive peptides

de novo analysis circumvents sequence databases by utilizing mass discrepancies among fragments to ascertain sequences. Prevalent database search engines comprise X!Tandem, Mascot, SEQUEST, MS-GFDB, MS-Fit, and OMSSA. In peptidomic search engine configurations, the enzyme type is frequently designated as "no enzyme" to optimize peptide identification. De novo tools, including Ustags, Peaks, PepNovo, Sherenga, DirecTag, and MS-Tag, are utilized separately [8]. Some tools, like OpenSea and DirecTag, integrate database and de novo approaches, enabling the identification of de novo-derived sequence tags and their comparison with protein databases.

Reversed-phase ultra-high-performance liquid chromatography (RP-UHPLC) separates molecules according to their hydrophobic interactions with the column material, whereas capillary electrophoresis (CE) employs an electric field to separate charged compounds. In CE, analyte ions are separated based on their electrophoretic mobility, which depends on the molecule of charge (*q*) and analyte of radius (r) wo methods offer strong complementarity [9], the extremely low flow rate of CE (typically under 20 nL/min) enables high separation performance and minimal ion suppression for polar substances that are challenging to resolve in liquid chromatography. Furthermore, the high separation efficiency of this technique ensures sensitive and reproducible identification of peptide peaks; according to current reports, a total of 106, 126, 89, and 113 peptides were respectively identified from 1 to 4 h simulated gastrointestinal digestion samples of *Crassostrea gigas* proteins using the CE-Q-TOF method [9]. After removing duplicate peptides, 425 unique peptides were obtained. Notably, the vast majority of peptides in the 4-h samples existed only in individual time points, with only one peptide being consistently present across all four time points.

4.4 Molecular Biological Information Prediction

Bioinformatics methods have been essential in forecasting the bioactivity of protein hydrolysates in several research contexts [10]. Numerous specialized databases, such as BIOPEP, PeptideDB, CAMP, APD2, and PepBank, provide as critical bioinformatics resources for the identification of bioactive peptide fragments in protein sequences. These resources help the categorization and analysis of bioactive peptides while providing predicted insights that assist in the identification and characterization of novel peptide sequences. Widely used online platforms, such as BIOPEP (http://www.uwm.edu.pl/biochemia/index.php/en/biopep) and ExPASy-PeptideCutter (http://web.Expasy.org/peptide_cutter), allow users to forecast peptide sequences that specific enzymes might release from target protein substrates [11]. The combination of virtual enzymatic digestion with bioactive peptide databases (such as BIOPEP) has enabled the development of enhanced hydrolysis methods. For example, calculations can be performed to determine the quantity of known bioactive peptides produced or the frequency with which bioactive peptides are generated along the protein chain. Computational simulations enable both single-enzyme and multienzyme hydrolysis models, allowing researchers to predict a wider spectrum of hydrolysates with bioactive properties. Table 4.2 summarizes the key bioinformatics resources and computational methods currently used for bioactivity prediction and peptide analysis.

A study utilized PeptideRanker scoring to assess peptide sequences in enzymatic hydrolysates of oyster proteins processed through various methods, including heating and homogenization. In the nonheated group, 53 peptides exhibited scores exceeding 0.4, accounting for 15.73% of the total identified peptides. After heat treatment at 100 °C, 16 peptides scored above 0.4, accounting for 24.62% of the total peptides. In proteins exposed to 100 MPa homogenization, 247 peptides were discovered, of which 34 peptides (13.77%) had scores exceeding 0.4. In a comparable manner, ultrasonic therapy at 900 W resulted in the identification of 271 peptides, of which 54 peptides (19.9%) achieved a score exceeding 0.4. Peptides with scores over 0.4 and comprising 10 amino acids or less were chosen for subsequent

Table 4.2 Bioinformatics databases and computing software

Database type	Name	Website	Function
Protein database	NCBI	https://www.ncbi.nlm.nih.gov/	Basic sequence information of proteins
	UniProtKB	http://www.uniprot.org/	Basic sequence and structural of proteins
	BIOPEP	http://www.uwm.edu.pl/biochemia/	Protein sequence database
Virtual enzyme hydrolysis database	PeptideCutter	http://web.expasy.org/peptide_cutter/	Virtual enzyme digestion
	BIOPEP	http://www.uwm.edu.pl/biochemia/index.php/en/biopep	Bioactive peptide database
	Enzyme Predictor	http://bioware.ucd.ie/~enzpred/Enzpred.php	Peptide enzymatic digestion database
Bioactive peptide database	BIOPEP	http://www.uwm.edu.pl/biochemia/index.php/en/biopep	Bioactive peptide database
	BitterDB	http://bitterdb.agri.huji.ac.il/bitterdb/	Bitter compound database
	EROP-Moscow database	http://erop.inbi.ras.ru	Bioactive peptide database
	PepBank	http://pepbank.mgh.harvard.edu/	Bioactive peptide database
Prediction of physicochemical properties	Expasy-Compute pI/Mw	http://web.expasy.org/compute_pi/	Hydrophilicity and instability calculator
	ProtParam	http://web.expasy.org/protparam/	Calculation of theoretical isoelectric point and molecular weight
	PepDraw	http://www.tulane.edu/~biochem/WW/PepDraw/	Calculation of net charge and hydrophobicity
Molecular simulation platform and algorithm	I-TASSER	https://zhanglab.ccmb.med.umich.edu/I-TASSER/	Protein structure and function prediction
	Discovery studio	–	Molecular docking, molecular dynamics
	Schrödinger	–	Molecular docking, molecular dynamics
	Gold	–	Molecular docking

study [11]. Bioinformatics has emerged as an essential and effective method for the identification of novel bioactive peptides. Recent studies emphasize its capacity to predict and analyze bioactive peptides derived from food proteins, providing insights into their potential activities through computational methods.

4.4.1 Activity Prediction

PeptideRanker is a bioactive peptide prediction server that utilizes a unique N-to-1 neural network model. Users can submit a list of peptides, which are graded based on their likelihood of having bioactivity. The server uses a default threshold of 0.5 and classifies any peptide with a predicted probability greater than this threshold as bioactive. Users can choose a higher threshold to reduce false positives, but this can affect the genuine positive rate. It is vital to note that PeptideRanker forecasts the likelihood of a peptide being bioactive without specifying which sort of bioactivity. Furthermore, the server for calculations and predictions is based on unaltered amino acid sequences. Post-translational changes like N-terminal acetylation, C-terminal amidation, or cyclization can improve a peptide's bioactivity and selectivity. As a result, peptides identified as potentially bioactive by PeptideRanker should undergo in vitro alterations to enhance their bioactivity.

4.4.2 Toxicity Prediction

Peptides exhibit potential as therapeutic agents for numerous disorders, rendering toxicity prediction a crucial step to guarantee their safety for subsequent research. The ToxinPred server is frequently utilized to forecast peptide toxicity and aid in the creation of nontoxic analogs via amino acid alterations. In the event that a peptide is identified as harmful, amino acid changes may be utilized to create analogs, which are subsequently tested and evaluated for favorable characteristics.

ToxinPred offers several key functionalities. (1) Peptide design: it enables the creation of peptide analogs through amino acid substitutions and predicts their toxicity. (2) Batch toxicity prediction: the tool can assess the toxicity of multiple peptides simultaneously. (3) Optimization: by submitting peptide sequences in FASTA format, users can optimize the sequence to achieve minimal, maximal, or desired toxicity based on position-specific scoring derived from quantitative matrices. This allows for the identification of peptides with the lowest or highest toxicity. (4) Physicochemical property prediction: the platform also provides insights into the physicochemical properties of peptides, aiding in their evaluation and refinement. By employing ToxinPred, researchers can efficiently design and refine peptides with minimal toxicity, paving the way for their therapeutic application.

4.4.3 Antimicrobial Activity Prediction

The Database of Antimicrobial Activity and Structure of Peptides (DBAASP) is a manually curated database. It was created to assist scientific researchers with information and analytical resources for developing antimicrobial compounds with a high therapeutic index. Antimicrobial peptides (AMPs) are ancient defense chemicals found in all life forms that play an important role in destroying invading pathogens such as bacteria, fungi, parasites, and viruses. Thus, AMPs are widely employed in medicine, food preservation, and agriculture. DBAASP informs users with the precise structure (chemistry, 3D) and antimicrobial activity of peptides against specified target species. The database contains information about ribosomal, nonribosomal, and synthetic peptides, which aids in the development of task-oriented new antibiotic designs with high-accuracy predictions, including the ability to forecast whether a peptide has antibacterial potential based on amino acid sequence. DBAASP gives information about synergistic activity. The data comprises the combined effect of a previously stored peptide in the database with another peptide or antimicrobial drug against a specific target strain, expressed as fractional inhibitory concentration (FICI) values. The search terms include website ID, structure, name, synthesis type, target group (Gram-positive or Gram-negative), sequence, and source (PubMed information). It can also show monomer information, changed amino acid information, and target species information, which can be utilized to create antimicrobial peptides and anticipate their characteristics and antimicrobial potency.

4.5 Summary

The field of seafood research is advancing swiftly; nevertheless, investigations focused on marine shellfish proteins and peptides remain comparatively scarce. The increasing recognition of the nutritional elements in seafood suggests that the conversion of shellfish nutrients into high-value peptide products will be a significant focus in marine-derived peptide research. The enzymatic hydrolysis of marine shellfish serves as a primary method for obtaining bioactive peptides. Advancements in peptide extraction, detection, and analysis are improving the throughput, accuracy, and feasibility of peptidomics. Peptidomics is set to progress with the creation of more rapid instruments that can separate and detect a greater number of peptide sequences in reduced time, alongside enhanced detectors that yield more comprehensive ion fragment data. Bioinformatics is increasingly recognized as a valuable tool in the peptide field and other chemical domains, especially in biochemistry related to fundamental research. Nonetheless, progress in these domains depends on multiple factors, including the purification and characterization of essential proteins serving as donors or receptors in biological processes; advancements in proteomics, particularly in food proteomics; molecular screening, identification of amino acid sequences, and structural characterization of specific biomarkers; clarification of the intricate mechanisms of bioactive peptides or proteins; and the ongoing development of bioinformatics tools to precisely calculate or predict donor–receptor interactions at the molecular level, including active sites, interacting amino acids, and interaction bonds. Advancements in biochemistry, chemistry, physical chemistry, computational chemistry, and X-ray crystallography will significantly enhance the application and development of peptide research.

References

1. Yu CP, Cha Y, Wu F, Fan WW, Xu XB, Du M. Effects of ball-milling treatment on mussel (*Mytilus edulis*) protein: structure, functional properties and *in vitro* digestibility. Int J Food Sci Technol. 2018;53(3):683–91.
2. Cao W, Feng Y, Tan C. Research progress of oyster protein and its peptide. Fine Spec Chem. 2020;28(4):4.
3. Guérard F, Decourcelle N, Sabourin C, Floch-Laizet C, Grel L, Floch P, Gourlay F, Délézir R, Jaouen P, Bourseau P. Recent developments of marine ingredients for food and nutraceutical applications: a review. J Sci Halieut Aquat. 2010;2:21–7.
4. Harnedy PA, FitzGerald RJ. Bioactive peptides from marine processing waste and shellfish: a review. J Funct Foods. 2012;4(1):6–24.
5. Afonso MD, Bórquez R. Review of the treatment of seafood processing wastewaters and recovery of proteins therein by membrane separation processes-prospects of the ultrafiltration of wastewaters from the fish meal industry. Desalination. 2002;142(1):29–45.
6. Dallas D, Guerrero A, Parker E, Robinson R, Gan J, German B, Barile D, Lebrilla C. Current peptidomics: applications, purification, identification, quantification, and functional analysis. Proteomics. 2015;15(5–6):1026–38.
7. Cheng S, Tu M, Liu H, Zhao G, Du M. Food-derived antithrombotic peptides: preparation, identification, and interactions with thrombin. Crit Rev Food Sci Nutr. 2019;59:1–15.
8. Tu M, Cheng S, Lu W, Du M. Advancement and prospects of bioinformatics analysis for studying bioactive peptides from food-derived protein: sequence, structure, and functions. TrAC Trends Anal Chem. 2018;105:7–17.
9. Chen H, Shi P, Fan F, Tu M, Xu Z, Xu X, Du M. Complementation of UPLC-Q-TOF-MS and CESI-Q-TOF-MS on identification and determination of peptides from bovine lactoferrin. J Chromatogr B. 2018;1084:150–7.
10. Ji L, Shao Y, Sun J, Shi L. Research on self-starting strategy of variable speed pumped storage units based on model predictive control. J Eng. 2017;2017(13):984–9.
11. Guo Z, Zhao F, Chen H, Tu M, Tao S, Wang Z, Wu C, He S, Du M. Heat treatments of peptides from oyster (*Crassostrea gigas*) and the impact on their digestibility and angiotensin I converting enzyme inhibitory activity. Food Sci Biotechnol. 2020;29(7):961–7.

Chapter 5
Marine Shellfish Peptides and Bone Health

Ming Du, Zhe Xu, Shuzhen Cheng, Zhihui Chang, and Ruibin Guo

Abstract Osteoporosis is a common illness that primarily affects elderly adults and postmenopausal women. In recent years, peptides produced from marine shellfish have attracted interest for their ability to promote bone health. This chapter examines the methodologies for the synthesis and identification of bone-promoting peptides derived from marine shellfish, encompassing virtual screening utilizing computational techniques and in vitro screening focused on bone-related indicators. Additional biochemical techniques, including flexible molecular docking and isothermal titration calorimetry, have been utilized to elucidate the activity and mechanisms of these bone-promoting peptides. The development of osteoblast and osteoclast models, coupled with investigations into signaling pathways, provides cellular-level data for comprehending the effects of the peptides. In animal models, methodologies, including as computed tomography and ultrasound imaging, have been employed to assess the effects of these peptides on osteoporosis. This chapter encapsulates the existing research advancements and provides novel perspectives for forthcoming osteoporosis therapies.

Keywords Osteoporosis · Marine shellfish peptide · Osteogenesis mechanism

Marine ecosystems exhibit significant diversity, offering a wide range of biological resources, notably seafood that is high in proteins and amino acids. Bioactive peptides obtained from marine shellfish demonstrate potential in enhancing bone formation and decreasing bone resorption. They are promising candidates for the

M. Du
College of Food Science and Engineering, Dalian Ocean University, Dalian, China

Z. Xu
Life Sciences, Dalian Minzu University, Dalian, China

S. Cheng (✉)
School of Food Science and Technology, Dalian Polytechnic University, Dalian, China

Z. Chang · R. Guo
Food Science and Engineering, Dalian Polytechnic University, Dalian, China

M. Du, S. Cheng (eds.), *Bioactive Proteins and Peptides from Marine Shellfish*,
https://doi.org/10.1007/978-981-95-3937-6_5

development of foods and drugs aimed at treating osteoporosis. This chapter presents an overview of the anti-osteoporosis properties of bioactive peptides derived from marine shellfish, detailing the processes of screening, identification, preparation, and the biological activity markers associated with osteogenic peptides. This text outlines the biochemical methods, cell models, and animal models employed to assess the osteogenic activity of these peptides. This chapter discusses the role of integrins in the screening and development of bioactive peptides derived from marine shellfish, thereby enhancing the breadth and depth of research in this area. In vitro cellular studies and in vivo animal models have demonstrated the efficacy of bioactive peptides derived from marine shellfish in the prevention of osteoporosis. These peptides potentially influence bone health through interactions with integrin RGD structures and the activation of signaling pathways, including BMP/Smads, MAPK, and OPG/RANKL/RANK. The process of shell formation in marine shellfish aligns with osteogenic mechanisms. Marine shellfish protein peptides represent a significant resource for the formulation of potential foods and pharmaceuticals aimed at enhancing bone growth.

5.1 Osteoporosis and Bone Density

5.1.1 Population with Osteoporosis

Osteoporosis is a systemic bone disease characterized by bone microstructure degradation, decreased bone density, and an increased fracture risk. Women who have gone through menopause are more sensitive to this disorder because of the decrease in estrogen levels, which is a key contributor to bone loss after menopause. In some Western countries, 13% of men and 40% of women over the age of 50 frequently develop fragility fractures [1]. Upon reaching the age of 40, the process of bone resorption often surpasses that of bone formation. This frequently includes periosteal growth, endosteal breakdown, increased cortical porosity, and a transformation of cortical bone to a more trabecular-like structure. The reduction in estrogen levels during menopause in women over 40 accelerates the aging process. Osteoporosis diagnosis involves several methods, one of which is the evaluation of bone mineral density (BMD) using dual-energy X-ray absorptiometry (DXA). Generally, BMD values are established at 2.5 standard deviations. Bone mineral density indicates the quantity of mineral content within a specific volume of bone, serving as a crucial measure of bone strength [2]. Calcium and phosphorus are the main components of bone minerals, and the more they are deposited in the bones, the stronger the bones will be. In clinical practice, when using bone density values, the *t*-score is often used to determine whether bone mineral density is normal, as there are differences in absolute values between different bone densitometers. The *t*-score is a relative value, and the usual reference range is between −1 and +1. $T < -2.5$ is considered abnormal. Bone density serves as a key indicator of bone health, highlighting the severity of osteoporosis and providing essential insights for assessing fracture risk. Aside from diagnosing osteoporosis, it is also useful for monitoring clinical outcomes and doing epidemiological research, making it an effective tool for predicting osteoporosis-related fractures.

5.1.2 *Pathogenesis of Osteoporosis*

Population aging is a global issue that poses a challenge to all countries and has a substantial impact on public health [3]. Many changes connected with aging raise the risk of chronic diseases. For instance, aging causes a loss in bone mass and strength, which leads to osteoporosis, one of the most common bone illnesses [4]. It is estimated that over 200 million people worldwide suffer from osteoporosis [5]. As the aging process increases, the prevalence of osteoporosis rises, and it has become a serious illness that endangers human health.

The body's bone metabolism is a dynamic and intricate cycle of continual renewal that includes two essential processes: bone formation by osteoblasts and bone destruction by osteoclasts. When the pace of bone breakdown exceeds the rate of bone synthesis, bone density often decreases, increasing the risk of osteoporosis. Osteoporosis is characterized by the breakdown of bone microstructure, reduced bone density, increased bone fragility, and is a chronic illness with a high fracture risk. During bone growth and development, osteoblasts (OBs) govern bone mineralization by secreting bone matrix and noncollagen, whereas osteoclasts (OCs) play a direct role in bone resorption [6]. Both bone formation and resorption are important and are directly and indirectly closely related to osteoporosis [7].

Bone is a dynamic and metabolically active tissue that perpetually remodels through the operations of osteoblasts and osteoclasts on the surfaces of osteoid and trabeculae. The two contrasting processes are termed bone remodeling or turnover. Due to its greater surface area, trabecular bone undergoes remodeling more frequently than cortical bone. Osteoblasts create new bone matrix, while osteoclasts degrade old bone matrix, ensuring a balance of bone formation and degradation. Every year, around 10% of the skeletal system is replaced, allowing bones to heal and adapt to mechanical stress [8]. A key aspect of bone remodeling is the regulation of calcium balance and metabolic activity [9, 10]. During childhood, bone development dominates the dynamic equilibrium of the bones, resulting in a rise in bone strength and size, with bone mass peaking between the ages of 20 and 30 [11–13]. At this point, bone resorption and formation are balanced, with the rate of resorption equal to the rate of formation.

5.2 Preparation and Identification of Bone Health-Promoting Peptides

Shellfish is gradually becoming an integral dietary item at the dinner table. In China, clam farming and harvesting are second only to fish aquaculture, with a total production of around 16.6 million tons in 2023. Current processing procedures generate 30–70% waste, with more than 40% of clam tissue thrown as garbage. This not only generates substantial trash, but it also pollutes the environment. Shellfish waste, comprising shells, viscera, and gonads, provides a lot of nutrients, especially protein. If these proteins are treated with enzymatic hydrolysis technology, they could be a lucrative source for industrial items like spices and functional foods. According to research, seafood consumption is positively connected with bone mass while being adversely correlated with the risk of osteoporosis [14, 15]. Consequently, shellfish proteins could serve as a possible functional food for the prevention of osteoporosis. In recent years, certain pharmaceutical and functional food development businesses have employed enzymatic hydrolysis technology to transform proteins from marine resources, such as fish and shellfish waste, into high-value goods. Shellfish protein hydrolysates are derived from shellfish and their by-products. Enzymatic hydrolysis can decompose shellfish proteins into peptides, including various amino acid units. This technology facilitates the efficient procurement of chemicals with advantageous biological functions for the human body, including amino acids and bioactive peptides. These hydrolysates possess high absorption efficiency and demonstrate remarkable bioactive properties, rendering them a significant resource for medications or functional foods.

Proteins' functional activity is determined by their amino acid sequence. Proteases hydrolyze proteins, releasing functionally active fragments. These fragments are significant sources of bioactive peptides with functional activities like antioxidant, antihypertensive, immunomodulatory, and osteogenic effects in addition to being essential sources of nitrogen and amino acids. According to recent studies, bioactive peptides from shellfish interact with proteins connected to bone in a specific way, showing promising bone-promoting properties.

5.2.1 Preparation of Bone Health-Promoting Peptides

To get shellfish protein hydrolysates, people usually use hydrolysis methods with acid, alkali, heat, or enzymes. However, thermal hydrolysis and acid–base hydrolysis can damage some amino acids and reduce nutritional value, which makes consumers less satisfied. For this reason, enzymatic hydrolysis is now the more common method for shellfish protein. By using food-grade enzymes to break proteins into specific peptides at specific sites, we can improve consumer satisfaction and make the preparation process easier to control. Choosing the right proteolytic enzymes is key to releasing osteogenic peptides from shellfish proteins.

The enzymes used in industry mainly originate from animals, plants, or microbes. Examples of common protein-digesting enzymes include bromelain (derived from pineapple stems), alkaline proteases, flavor-enhancing enzymes, pancreatic digestive enzymes, pancreatic enzyme complexes, gastric digestive enzymes, fungal proteases, pancreatic serine proteases, rennet, neutral proteases, and papaya-derived

Table 5.1 Shellfish peptides for osteoporosis

Source	Peptide sequence	Functional activity
Crassostrea gigas protein hydrolysates	YRGDVVPK	Promote proliferation of osteoblasts [14]
Mytilus edulis protein hydrolysates	LGKDQVRT	Promote proliferation and differentiation of osteoblasts [15]
	YPRKDETGAERT	Promote proliferation and differentiation of osteoblasts [16]
	IEELEEELEAER	Promotes osteoblast growth and inhibits osteoclast proliferation [17]
	PIISVYWK	Promoting differentiation of bone marrow mesenchymal stem cells into osteoblasts [16]
	FSVVPSPK	Promoting differentiation of bone marrow mesenchymal stem cells into osteoblasts [18]
Ark shell protein hydrolysates	AWLNH	Promoting differentiation of bone mesenchymal stem cells into osteoblasts [19]
	PHDL	Promoting differentiation of bone mesenchymal stem cells into osteoblasts [19]

enzymes. When using enzymes to break down proteins, it is important to focus on hydrolysis efficiency. Temperature and pH have the biggest effect on how well the reaction works. Further details on the various types of proteases and the production of shellfish-derived osteogenic peptides can be found in Chap. 3. There are numerous sources of shellfish-derived osteogenic active peptides, including oysters, mussels, and ark shells. Table 5.1 shows some peptides with strong osteogenic activity.

5.2.2 Screening and Identification of Bone Health-Promoting Peptides

Scientists assess the osteogenic potential of bioactive peptides through specific tests. These tests measure the peptides' ability to stimulate osteoblast growth and maturation. They also measure the ability to inhibit osteoclast formation and activity. Common assessment methods include two main approaches. One approach is quantifying bone mineral density in animal models. The other is conducting human clinical studies. However, these traditional assessment techniques have a major drawback. They often require a significant amount of time and resources. This characteristic makes them less feasible for initial large-scale screening purposes. Therefore, a summary of these methods has been created. This summary helps facilitate the rapid screening and identification of peptides with potential osteogenic activity.

5.2.2.1 Virtual Screening Based on Computational Algorithms

The bioactivity of bioactive peptides depends on their amino acid sequence. Currently, several online servers exist for predicting peptide structures. These servers include Pep-Fold, PEPstrMOD, Protinfo, Hmmstr/Rosetta, and I-Tasser. Researchers can use software tools like Discovery Studio, Sybyl, and ArgusLab. These tools help predict peptide structures. They also enable further refinement of these structures. The refinement process involves energy minimization and molecular dynamics simulations [20, 21]. Scientists use Discovery Studio software to forecast molecular configurations. The software employs force field principles. These principles include a collection of parameters and formulas. Researchers apply them in molecular mechanics computations. The process of molecular docking has a specific design. It estimates the interaction strength between small molecules and receptor proteins. It also identifies their interaction sites. Researchers examine the structure–activity relationship of bioactive peptides and proteins. This examination helps identify shellfish protein peptides. These peptides may exhibit osteoinductive properties.

Integrins act as crucial regulatory proteins in cellular processes. They represent a class of heterodimeric membrane receptors. These receptors consist of distinct α and β chains. Integrins function as bidirectional signaling receptors. They possess specialized domains. These domains interact with extracellular matrix components. This interaction influences cellular growth and movement. The integrin family includes 18 distinct α chain variants. It also includes eight β chain variants. These variants allow for the formation of 24 unique heterodimeric receptor combinations. The combinations form through various subunit pairings [22]. According to their molecular recognition patterns, integrins are predominantly divided into two groups: those that interact with the tripeptide sequence Arg-Gly-Asp and those that recognize distinct molecular motifs. Figure 5.1 demonstrates that non-RGD receptors can

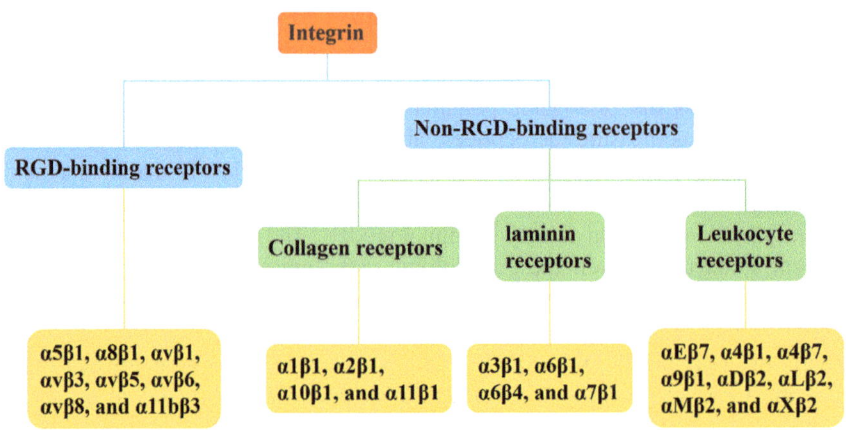

Fig. 5.1 Classification of integrins. Integrins are categorized into RGD-binding receptors and non-RGD-binding receptors

be divided into three main categories: immune cell receptors (αDβ2, αEβ7, αLβ2, αMβ2, αXβ2, α4β1, α4β7, α9β1), collagen-binding receptors (α1β1, α2β1, α10β1, α11β1), and laminin-binding receptors (α3β1, α6β1, α7β1). Meanwhile, RGD receptors primarily consist of αvβ1, αvβ3, αvβ5, αvβ6, αvβ8, α5β1, α8β1, and αIIbβ3 [23]. Bioactive peptides are characteristic protein fragments. They can interact or bind with specific receptors. This interaction or binding helps them express activity. It also allows them to regulate physiological functions. α5β1 integrin heterodimers have an important presence. They not only upregulate phospho-RUNX2 levels. They also initiate focal adhesion kinase signaling. This signaling subsequently triggers two cascades. These cascades are the extracellular signal-regulated kinase cascade and the mitogen-activated protein kinase cascade [24]. Additionally, it can induce the differentiation of osteoblasts. Integrin αvβ3 can activate the Shc and FAK pathways [25]. Furthermore, studies have found that integrin-RGD complexes can support and participate in growth factor-induced cell cycle processes.

The β1 integrin subunit and the peptide sequence RVYFFKGKQYWE bind specifically, and this specific binding substantially enhances the multiplication of bone-forming cells. Integrin α5β1 can improve three key processes in osteoblasts: adhesion, proliferation, and differentiation. However, some bioactive peptides act differently by interfering with integrin αvβ3, which disrupts the cytoskeleton of osteoclasts and thereby inhibits osteoclast proliferation. Therefore, the interaction between bioactive peptides, integrins α5β1 or αvβ3, and the extracellular matrix plays a crucial role as it affects the proliferation and differentiation of osteoblasts or osteoclasts. Peptides with potential osteogenic activity interact with integrins α5β1 or αvβ3, and this interaction is considered an indicator that shows whether the peptides promote osteoblasts or inhibit osteoclasts. This section will list relevant parameters of integrins α5β1 and αvβ3 that help screen for osteogenic active peptides, as shown in Table 5.2. After researchers determine how osteogenic active peptides interact with integrins, some of these peptides can be used as factors that aid in bone defect repair. Integrins belong to the family of cell adhesion receptors and can regulate two important aspects: the localization and activity of proteases, and cell adhesion and proliferation. Corresponding bioactive peptides, such as osteogenic active peptides, work effectively by interacting with integrins, and this interaction promotes various cellular functions including proliferation and differentiation. The preparation methods for integrins and osteogenic peptides are described above, and

Table 5.2 Two integrins used for screening bone peptides

Category	αVβ3	α5β1
Specific PDB number	1L5G	3VI4
Identification method	X-RAY DIFFRACTION	X-RAY DIFFRACTION
Resolution	3.20 Å	2.90 Å
Total structure weight	187.43 kDa	339.88 kDa
Atom count	11,700	22,882
Unique protein chains	3	5
R-value free	0.328 (depositor)	0.275 (depositor)

these substances can accelerate the healing of bone defects. The evaluation methods mentioned earlier have two benefits: they reduce costs and increase speed, and once verification is completed, these methods and peptides can be applied quickly.

5.2.2.2 In Vitro Screening Based on Bone-Related Biomarkers

Bone formation biomarkers indicate various phases in the bone formation process (Table 5.3). Key enzymes, including bone-specific alkaline phosphatase (Bone ALP), serum alkaline phosphatase (S-ALP), and total alkaline phosphatase (T-ALP), are found on cell surfaces. Tissue nonspecific genes are primarily active in bones and the liver, while tissue-specific genes are expressed in the placenta, intestines, and germline enzymes. Nontissue-specific and tissue-specific alkaline phosphatase isoforms are encoded by identical genetic sequences, but they demonstrate distinct biological characteristics. This difference arises from the differential processing and

Table 5.3 Biomarkers of osteoporosis

Category	Source	Bone formation marker (BFM)/bone resorption marker (BRM)	Abbreviation
Alkaline phosphatase	Bones, liver, placenta, intestines, kidneys	BFM	ALP
Bone-derived alkaline phosphatase	Osteoblasts	BFM	Bone ALP
Procollagen I carbon end extension bone peptide	Bones, skin, tendons and ligaments, arterial walls	BFM	PICP
Procollagen I nitrogen end extension bone peptide	Bones, skin, tendons and ligaments, arterial walls	BFM	PINP
Osteocalcin	Osteoblasts	BFM	OC
Tartrate-resistant acid phosphatase 5b	Osteoblast	BRM	TRACP5b
C-terminal cross-linked terminal peptide of type I collagen	Bones, teeth, skin	BRM	CTX
Nitrogen-terminal cross-linked terminal peptide of type I collagen	Bones, teeth, skin	BRM	NTX
Carbon terminal cross-linked terminal peptide of type I collagen produced by metalloproteinases	Bones, joints, skin, vascular walls	BRM	ICTP
Deoxypyridinoline	Bones, teeth, skin	BRM	DPD
Pyridinoline	Bones, cartilage, teeth, skin, tendons, blood vessels	BRM	PYD

alteration of their sugar chain structures [26]. ALP is present on the surface of osteoblasts in the bone. It is then solubilized and released into the bloodstream. For this reason, changes in the bone and liver can affect serum ALP levels. In healthy adults, more than half of the alkaline phosphatase comes from bones and is released into the serum. Thus, serum alkaline phosphatase often serves as a marker of bone turnover. However, it still lacks specificity and sensitivity in some cases. Bone ALP is being used more and more to improve measurement sensitivity. But a 15–20% overlap remains in the analyses of liver and bone ALP [27]. Osteocalcin, also known as bone Gla protein, is a noncollagenous matrix protein in bone. It is a low molecular weight protein. Osteoblasts, preosteoblasts, mast chondrocytes, and odontoblasts express this protein. Moreover, osteocalcin contains three gamma-carboxylated glutamate moieties. These moieties show significant binding affinity toward calcium ions. The calcium ions are within the crystalline structure of bone mineral [28]. Hydroxyapatite is the main inorganic component of human and animal bones. Circulating osteocalcin represents a measurable fraction of this bone-specific protein, while the remainder becomes incorporated into the mineralized bone structure. This characteristic makes blood osteocalcin levels a valuable indicator for assessing bone formation rates and osteoblastic function. Serum osteocalcin has three components: one-third consists of small fragments, one-third consists of mid-molecule fragments (comprising residues 1–43), and one-third is intact osteocalcin [29]. Osteocalcin can also be released during bone resorption and is rapidly degraded once it enters circulation. Some osteocalcin fragments can be found in the kidneys and liver. Urine osteocalcin levels do not affect the synthesis of type I collagen during bone formation; however, they are associated with the process of bone degeneration. Extracellular production of type I collagen involves the cleavage of two terminal peptides prior to fibril assembly. These peptides promote the helical formation of collagen, and their cleavage fragments—C-terminal (PICP) and N-terminal (PINP) peptides—are detectable in the blood. Thus, PINP and PICP concentrations provide a quantitative measure of type I collagen production. Type I collagen is found in bone and soft tissue, but it is more rapidly transformed in bone, which makes serum PICP and PINP levels a reliable marker of bone-specific collagen metabolism.

Biomarkers of bone destruction include tartrate-resistant acid phosphatases, terminal peptide fragments of type I collagen, matrix metalloproteinase-derived collagen fragments, pyridine cross-links, and the bone-specific protein osteocalcin. Among these, TRACP5b is a phosphatase active at low pH, and it is mainly found in bone resorption cells, tissue macrophages, and their precursors. Two forms of TRACP exist in the circulatory system: macrophage-derived TRACP5a and osteoclast-specific TRACP5b, each with different pH-dependent activity profiles. The physiological role of TRACP5b secreted by osteoclasts is not fully understood. This enzyme is internalized through vesicle transport and involved in the breakdown of the bone matrix by promoting the production of reactive oxygen species in intracellular compartments, making it a reliable indicator of osteoclast activity and bone turnover.

Since kidney function has little effect on TRACP5b, food intake does not affect circulating levels of TRACP5b. However, TRACP5b is highly stable in serum [30]. Collagen has high structural stability due to its intramolecular and intermolecular cross-linking. In bones, deoxypyridinoline (DPD) and pyridinoline (PYD) form these cross-links. When collagen degrades, the cross-links between DPD and PYD are released. PYD is predominant in collagen, while DPD—more abundant in dentin and bone—is considered a bone-characteristic cross-link. This cross-linking is degraded in the kidneys. Both free cross-links and those bound to short collagen peptides can be measured in serum or urine. Type I collagen cross-linked telopeptides (ICTP) include cross-linked C-terminal telopeptides (CTX) and cross-linked N-terminal telopeptides (NTX). Different pathways of collagen breakdown produce different fragments: NTX and CTX are produced by cathepsin K, while ICTP is produced by matrix metalloproteinases [31]. CTX exists in two forms: non-isomerized α-CTX and isomerized β-CTX. Bone tissue aging correlates with the isomerization process of collagen crosslinks. This correlation enables the evaluation of aged bone degradation through the quantification of β-isomerized crosslinked telopeptides. Among various analytical approaches, β-CTX-1 measurement has emerged as a predominant technique for assessing bone collagen degradation products.

5.3 Analysis of Activity and Mechanism

5.3.1 Biochemical Methods

The biochemical assay method for osteogenic peptide activity primarily involves two key steps. These steps are predicting and validating the interactions between bioactive peptides and functional proteins.

5.3.1.1 Flexible Molecular Docking

The flexible molecular docking technique allows researchers to analyze several aspects of RGD/integrin interactions (Fig. 5.2). These aspects include the molecular mechanism, location, type, and energy of the interactions. Under the CHARMm force field, the "-CDOCKER ENERGY" parameter can predict the docking energy score of RGD/integrin. This score is used to analyze the binding affinity between the molecules [32]. The interaction energy between integrin α5β1 and the native RGD fragment is 116.249 kcal/mol. The "-CDOCKER ENERGY" interaction energy between integrin α5β1 and the PIE peptide is 191.364 kcal/mol. The interacting sites between integrin α5β1 (PDB: 3VI4) and native RGD include GLU320, ASP259, GLU229, SER227, ASP22, ASN224, LEU225, CYS187, PHE187, LYS182, SER134, and SER132. The interacting sites between integrin α5β1 and the

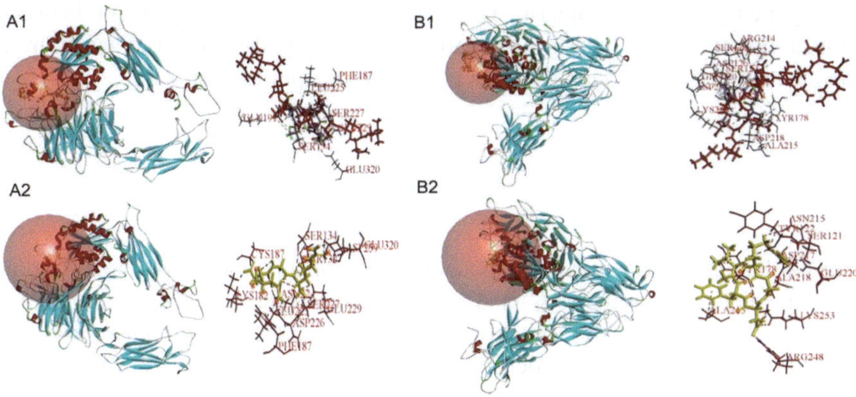

Fig. 5.2 Interaction between the PIE peptide and 3VI4 (**a**) and 1L5G (**b**) using flexible molecular docking technology. (1) Interaction between the PIE and integrin. (2) Interaction between native RGD and integrin

PIE peptide are GLU320, SER134, GLU229, SER227, LEU225, ASN224, GLN191, and PHE187. The amino acid interaction sites between integrin α5β1 (PDB: 3VI4) and the PIE peptide—including GLU320, GLU229, SER227, LEU225, ASN224, PHE187, and SER134—are similar to those of native RGD [16]. The peptide YGRDVVPK and peptide YPRKDETGAERT have more binding sites with integrin (PDB: 3VI4) and exhibit stronger affinity than native RGD, demonstrating osteogenic activity [17]. Therefore, osteogenic peptides can be screened through the analysis of three key factors. These factors are the interaction sites, forces, and energy between integrin and either the peptide or the native RGD active site.

5.3.1.2 Isothermal Titration Calorimetry

This method determines two key aspects: the interaction between osteogenic peptides and integrins, and their stoichiometric ratio. It achieves this by measuring four parameters of the entire reaction system containing peptides and proteins during titration. These parameters are the binding constant (K), stoichiometry (n), enthalpy change (ΔH), and entropy change (ΔS) [33].

5.3.1.3 Macromolecular Interaction Instrument

I In addition to isothermal titration calorimetry, macromolecular interaction analysis is another method used to verify the interaction between peptides and proteins. The macromolecular interaction instrument employs rapid labeling detection technology to perform molecular dynamics analysis on biological interference signals. The process involves two main steps: first, a biotinylation reagent is used to biotinylate the peptide; then, an SA sensor is used to measure the interaction between the biotinylated peptide and integrin. This method determines the interaction between biomacromolecules by measuring the affinity constant (Kd), which is obtained from the interaction between labeled target proteins and peptides [34].

5.3.2 *Cellular Model*

Normal human bone tissue exhibits active metabolism. Continuous bone resorption—mediated by osteoclasts—and bone formation—mediated by osteoblasts—occur on the trabecular surface and within the bone matrix. When bone resorption exceeds bone formation, bone density decreases. Excessively low bone density can lead to the disruption of bone microstructure and increased bone fragility. These are characteristic features of osteoporosis, a chronic disease that increases the risk of fractures. Therefore, the active cell model methods related to osteogenic peptides mainly include two types: osteoblast models and osteoclast models.

5.3.2.1 Osteoblast Model

The osteoblast model includes the assessment of two key processes: osteoblast proliferation and differentiation. There are various methods to measure osteoblast proliferation. For example, the osteogenic activity of peptides can be determined by culturing MC3T3-E1 cells and conducting a CCK-8 assay. Additionally, flow cytometry can be employed to analyze osteoblast cell cycle progression, which helps ascertain their proliferation status by examining the state of cells at different stages. Furthermore, the expression of signaling protein RNA can be measured using RT-Q-PCR, and the expression levels of signal transduction proteins can be determined through Western blotting; these techniques help verify the signaling pathways through which osteogenic peptides affect osteoblasts. In terms of osteoblast differentiation, biomarkers produced during osteoblast culture—such as alkaline phosphatase—can be measured. Osteoblast alkaline phosphatase can be quantified using specific assay kits, or osteoblasts can be stained to determine the amount of alkaline phosphatase present.

5.3.2.2 Osteoclast Model

The osteoclast model includes assays for two key functions: inhibiting osteoclast proliferation and differentiation. One method to evaluate osteoclast viability involves stimulating the transformation of RAW264.7 cells into osteoclasts, followed by an MTT assay to assess how osteogenic peptides influence the suppression of osteoclast proliferation. Similar to the osteoblast model, flow cytometry can also be used to determine the growth cycle of osteoclasts, thereby identifying their inhibition status. Osteoclasts are also involved in several signaling pathways; these can be examined by measuring the RNA expression levels of signaling proteins using RT-Q-PCR and detecting the expression levels of signal transduction proteins through Western blotting, which helps verify the signaling pathways affected by osteogenic peptides in osteoclasts.

For assessing osteoclast differentiation, biomarkers produced during the induction and culture of osteoclasts can be used, such as tartrate-resistant acid phosphatase (TRAP). This enzyme's activity can be quantified using specialized kits, and TRAP levels can also be assessed through staining the osteoclasts.

5.3.2.3 Signal Transduction Pathways in Bone Metabolism

The signaling pathways involved in bone metabolism mainly consist of four key pathways: the Wnt/β-catenin, RANK/RANKL/OPG, BMP/Smads, and Notch pathways. These pathways can directly affect bone marrow mesenchymal stem cells, thereby regulating the proliferation and maturation of bone cells. They can also transmit signals by regulating the communication between osteoblasts and osteoclasts. The Wnt/β-catenin, RANK/RANKL/OPG, and Notch pathways all function via glycogen synthase kinase 3 (GSK3). GSK3 contains two independently encoded isoform genes located on chromosomes: GSK3α and GSK3β. As a key regulator of stem cell pluripotency, GSK3 is a highly conserved Ser/Thr kinase belonging to the CMGC family (CDK, MAPK, GSK3, CLK) and is expressed across all tissues [15].

1. Wnt/β-Catenin Pathway

Wnt proteins are secreted glycoproteins that act through local signaling mechanisms to control cell proliferation and development. The primary receptor for the Wnt signaling pathway is low-density lipoprotein receptor-related protein 5, which is closely linked to human skeletal development. The Wnt/β-catenin signaling pathway contributes to increased bone mass through various means: promoting osteoblast proliferation, inducing osteoblast differentiation, inhibiting osteoblast apoptosis, and suppressing the differentiation of adipocytes and chondrocytes [35]. An elevated OPG/RANKL ratio, for example, stimulates Wnt/β-catenin signaling, thereby suppressing the formation of osteoclasts. Different Wnt proteins play distinct roles during bone development: Wnt7b induces osteoblast differentiation, while Wnt10b expression correlates with bone density and osteocalcin levels. Additionally, bone morphogenetic protein-2 can modulate the expression levels of Wnt1, Wnt4, and Wnt14 within osteoblasts [36].

2. RANK/RANKL/OPG Pathway

The RANK/RANKL/OPG pathway is a crucial communication route among bone cells, and its modulation significantly impacts bone remodeling. This pathway explains how the osteoblast lineage controls the differentiation and function of osteoclasts, involving three key components: RANK, a receptor present on hematopoietic precursor cells (osteoclast precursors); RANKL, a polypeptide expressed by osteoblasts and released in a soluble form; and osteoprotegerin (OPG), a decoy receptor secreted by osteoblasts. Osteoclast precursor cells differentiate into mature osteoclasts only when RANK binds to RANKL. Numerous hormones and cytokines influence physiological processes by regulating this signaling pathway [37]. Imbalances in the levels of RANKL and OPG can interfere with bone remodeling, highlighting the importance of therapeutic strategies aimed at correcting this imbalance. Osteoblasts integrate and analyze physiological and pathological signals from the environment to regulate the production of RANKL/OPG, thereby controlling bone resorption. When the expression of RANKL exceeds that of OPG, bone resorption increases, which can predispose individuals to skeletal diseases such as osteoporosis, Paget's disease, and metastatic bone cancer [38].

3. BMP/Smads Pathway

The role of bone morphogenetic protein (BMP) is to serve as a bone formation signal that mediates the bone formation pathway. BMP activates its target cells by binding to both type I and type II receptors, forming a receptor complex. The type II BMP receptor, which is always phosphorylated, activates the type I receptor through phosphorylation. This, in turn, triggers the phosphorylation of R-Smads 1/5/8—a key step in the BMP signaling pathway. Although the signaling pathways of BMP and TGF-β share similarities, such as receptor activation and the involvement of R-Smads, they differ in the specific receptor types and R-Smad proteins involved [39]. BMP signaling primarily involves Smad 1/5/8, while TGF-β signals mainly through Smad 2/3. Additionally, non-Smad signaling pathways are also activated by BMP and TGF-β receptors. For example, BMP receptors can influence the transcription of p38 and ERK in the MAPK pathway. The regulation of BMP's pleiotropic signaling responses, which control various physiological functions, is tightly controlled and, together with various regulatory mechanisms, forms a complex biological network [40].

4. Notch Pathway

In bone tissue, the differentiation and activity of osteoblasts and osteoclasts depend on the activation of Notch signaling. Notch is a membrane-bound protein with four receptor types: Notch1, Notch2, Notch3, and Notch4 [41]. These receptors interact with ligands to regulate various cellular functions. Ligand binding activates Notch signaling, leading to receptor cleavage and the release of the Notch intracellular domain (NICD), which then enters the nucleus. Inside the nucleus, NICD associates with CBF-1/RBP-Jκ, CSL, and MAML proteins to initiate gene transcription. Notch signaling plays a role in bone marrow mesenchymal cell differentiation by preventing commitment to osteoblast and chondrocyte lineages while promoting OPG expression, which suppresses osteoclastogenesis. In humans, altered Notch signaling is linked to skeletal disorders such as Alagille syndrome, spondylocostal dysostosis, and Hajdu–Cheney syndrome, with JAG1 and Notch2 mutations affecting bone mineral density. Additionally, overexpression of Notch1 correlates with osteosarcoma and breast cancer skeletal invasiveness. In conclusion, Notch signaling inhibits skeletal cell differentiation and is involved in skeletal disease pathogenesis during both development and postnatal stages [42].

5.3.3 *Animal Model*

5.3.3.1 Computed Tomography Diagnostics

Measuring bone mineral density (BMD) is among the most effective methods for characterizing osteoporosis. Currently, there are three main well-established models of osteoporosis in research: castration (removal of ovaries or testes), intragastric administration of retinoic acid, and glucocorticoid intramuscular injection. Additionally, there are other modeling methods, such as the low-calcium diet model and the parathyroid hormone model. Regardless of the modeling method used, bone mineral density—which characterizes the activity of osteogenic peptides—is determined by Micro-CT. Micro-CT can further assess bone tissue health by measuring related parameters, including bone volume (BV), tissue volume (TV), the ratio of bone volume to tissue volume (BV/TV), trabecular thickness (Tb.Th), trabecular pattern factor (Tb.Pf), trabecular separation (Tb.Sp), trabecular number (Tb.N), and bone mineral density (BMD).

5.3.3.2 Bone Tissue Sectioning

Bone tissue is made into slices, and through image analysis, the morphology and density of the bones are observed and calculated to diagnose osteoporosis in a more intuitive manner. However, preparing bone tissue slices is quite challenging. Since the hardness of bone depends on its calcium salt content, bone tissue must be decalcified and softened before slicing, which increases the difficulty of pathological diagnosis. The commonly used method for bone tissue decalcification is the acid immersion method. However, this method has drawbacks such as long decalcification time and corrosion risk, which can easily lead to damage to the bone tissue structure. In bone tissue slices, trabecular number is typically determined through staining to assess the presence of osteoporosis.

5.3.3.3 Ultrasonic Detection Method

The ultrasound testing method uses specialized ultrasound transducers to emit ultrasonic waves from the bone being tested. After passing through the bone and soft tissue, the method measures ultrasound wave velocity and attenuation rate to perform non-acoustic calculations, which are then compared to standard values for diagnosis. This is a new, noninvasive method for diagnosing osteoporosis, offering advantages such as ease of operation, nonradioactivity, cost-effectiveness, and safety. However, compared to the X-ray absorptiometry method, its accuracy still needs improvement.

5.3.3.4 Determination of Biomarkers in Serum

The biochemical marker detection method has the advantages of being noninvasive and highly sensitive, making it an effective approach for evaluating bone metabolism. This method primarily involves detecting the levels of markers in animal urine and blood, such as calcium, phosphorus, vitamin D, parathyroid hormone, bone alkaline phosphatase, and osteocalcin, to understand the basic condition of bone metabolism. This helps in the differential diagnosis of primary and secondary osteoporosis.

5.3.3.5 Commonly Used Osteoporosis Animal Model

1. Ovariectomy Model

The ovary is an organ responsible for oocyte development and hormone production. The hypothalamus and pituitary release gonadotropins, which regulate the ovary's control of FSH and LH. Hypothalamic GnRH regulates LH release in pulses, and through positive feedback, LH triggers the surge needed for ovulation. In the ovary, inhibin provides dual negative feedback to regulate FSH, while sex hormones, especially estrogen and progesterone, also play a role in FSH regulation. Estrogen is essential for bone metabolism and homeostasis, and its deficiency is a key factor in osteoporosis development. Bilateral ovariectomy in female rats is a well-established animal model that successfully simulates osteoporosis caused by estrogen deficiency. This model also helps study how estrogen deficiency damages other human systems. Estrogen is a key hormone that regulates bone metabolism in the body. After mice undergo ovariectomy, the resulting estrogen deficiency accelerates bone turnover, intensifies bone metabolism, reduces osteoblast numbers, and promotes osteoclast activation. These changes lead to lower bone density, damaged bone structure, and a higher risk of osteoporosis. In the ovariectomized model, mouse bone marrow mesenchymal stem cells lose much of their ability to promote bone formation, while periodontitis becomes more severe. This is linked to reduced osteogenic capacity and proliferation of periodontal ligament fibroblasts after estrogen deficiency.

2. Intragastric Retinoic Acid Model

After model rats received oral administration of retinoic acid, several changes were observed. Their food intake decreased significantly, and they lost marked weight. They became less active, with visible signs like arched backs and raised fur. The model rats showed remarkable alterations in cancellous bone mass and trabecular structure in the proximal tibia. These included a notable decline in trabecular area percentage and density, along with widened trabecular spacing. Histomorphometric analysis of bone tissue sections from the model animals revealed a marked decrease in cortical bone area at the tibial midshaft. This was accompanied by an expansion of the bone marrow cavity. The percentage of bone resorption perimeter on the endosteal surface increased significantly. This perimeter reflects the activity and function of osteoclasts. This model has several advantages. It is easy to develop, with a brief modeling period and a high success rate. It effectively replicates typical osteoporosis characteristics in animals, making it suitable for drug administration studies.

Retinoic acid is a derivative of vitamin A. It has pharmacological effects similar to vitamin A. Clinically, it is mainly used to treat various dermatological diseases. But it has a side effect: it can cause osteoporosis. Earlier research has shown that retinoic acid stimulates osteoclast activity. This stimulation leads to enhanced bone resorption. However, it does not suppress osteoblast function. Nor does it have a significant impact on bone formation and matrix mineralization. As a result, the body's bone remodeling process gets disrupted. It favors the breakdown of bone tissue over its regeneration. This eventually leads to osteoporosis in animals. The pathological morphology changes in this osteoporosis model are highly characteristic. Under the microscope, one can see trabecular sparsity, cortical bone thinning, and an enlarged bone marrow cavity. But because of how the model is established, it may cause gonadal damage in model animals. It may also lead to compensatory hypertrophy of the spleen and adrenal glands. For these reasons, it is less practical for research than the ovariectomy-induced osteoporosis model.

3. Glucocorticoid Intramuscular Injection Model

After rats received intramuscular injections of glucocorticoids, they showed notable weight loss. Microscopic examination of bone tissue sections revealed several changes. The trabecular area decreased, trabecular spacing widened, and mineral deposition and bone formation rates declined. The mechanism behind the glucocorticoid-induced osteoporosis animal model mainly involves supraphysiological doses of corticosteroids. These doses inhibit osteoblast activity, leading to reduced bone formation. Furthermore, glucocorticoids interfere with the regulation of calcium, phosphorus, vitamin D, and parathyroid hormone. This interference accelerates the process of bone breakdown, tipping the balance toward resorption rather than formation. As a result, this disruption causes a decrease in bone density, ultimately leading to osteoporosis. This model has positive significance for studying glucocorticoid-induced secondary osteoporosis in humans.

4. Other Models

In addition to the three common animal models for osteoporosis mentioned above, there are several other models used for specific research purposes.

Orchidectomized Rat Model In this model, male rats aged 4–6 months undergo orchidectomy. This procedure leads to rapid bone mass loss. The reason is that the rats fail to reach their peak bone mass. After testicular removal, the rate of bone metabolism turnover increases. Osteoporosis in this model mainly impacts the trabecular bone. However, these osteoporotic changes can be reversed with androgen replacement therapy.

Disuse Osteoporosis Model Bone mass and metabolism in animal limbs are closely related to several factors. These include load-bearing, muscle strength stimulation, and neuromuscular nourishment. Common methods to replicate this model involve specific procedures on one side of the animal. They include mechanical fixation, suspension, and surgical removal of the sciatic nerve, knee muscle, or Achilles tendon. The mechanisms by which disuse leads to osteoporosis are not entirely the same. So, results from one disuse model cannot be applied to others. Bone mass usually recovers after disuse factors are removed. But the recovery time is much longer than the time taken to induce the model. Currently, researchers recommend combining disuse models with either ovariectomy or orchidectomy for senile osteoporosis research. The former simulates reduced physical activity in the elderly. The latter simulates osteoporosis caused by declining gonadal function.

Low Calcium Diet-Induced Osteoporosis Model Long-term feeding of a low calcium diet can cause osteoporosis in animals. Blood acts as the body's calcium reservoir. It allows calcium to be mobilized or stored as needed. Parathyroid hormone and calcitonin regulate serum calcium levels. They keep these levels within a normal range. Parathyroid hormone promotes the transfer of calcium from bone into the bloodstream. This process increases blood calcium levels. In contrast, calcitonin inhibits bone resorption. It also stops calcium from moving from bone to blood.

5.4 Summary

Food protein hydrolysates and bioactive peptides have immeasurable potential as raw materials for future foods. Using bioinformatics to predict osteogenic active peptides in enzymatic hydrolysates helps understand the peptides' active groups at the molecular scale. This greatly reduces time and experimental costs. For subsequent processing to prepare functional peptides, advanced instruments and techniques are used. These include purification systems, mass spectrometry, bioinformatics, crystal purification systems, protein interaction analyzers, and micro-computed tomography. In conclusion, this chapter aims to provide a theoretical foundation. It focuses on developing shellfish-based foods to prevent osteoporosis by studying the mechanisms. These mechanisms are related to how shellfish-derived osteogenic peptides prevent osteoporosis.

References

1. Melton LJ 3rd, Chrischilles EA, Cooper C, Lane AW, Riggs BL. How many women have osteoporosis? JBMR Anniversary Classic. JBMR, Volume 7, Number 9, 1992. J Bone Miner Res. 2005;20(5):886–92.
2. Vestergaard P. Discrepancies in bone mineral density and fracture risk in patients with type 1 and type 2 diabetes—a meta-analysis. Osteoporos Int. 2007;18(4):427–44.

3. Shapses SA, Pop LC, Wang Y. Obesity is a concern for bone health with aging. Nutr Res. 2017;39:1–13.
4. Siddique N, O'Donoghue M, Casey MC, Walsh JB. Malnutrition in the elderly and its effects on bone health – a review. Clin Nutr ESPEN. 2017;21:31–9.
5. Reginster J-Y, Burlet N. Osteoporosis: a still increasing prevalence. Bone. 2006;38(2 Suppl 1):S4–9.
6. Cann CE, Martin MC, Genant HK, Jaffe RB. Decreased spinal mineral content in amenorrheic women. JAMA. 1984;251(5):626–9.
7. Ming D, Zhe X, Hui C, Fengjiao F, Pujie S, Di W. Chapter 27 – Food-derived osteogenic peptides towards osteoporosis. In: Biologically active peptides. Academic Press; 2021. p. 665–88.
8. Manolagas SC. Birth and death of bone cells: basic regulatory mechanisms and implications for the pathogenesis and treatment of osteoporosis. Endocr Rev. 2000;21(2):115–37.
9. Parfitt AM. Targeted and nontargeted bone remodeling: relationship to basic multicellular unit origination and progression. Bone. 2002;30(1):5–7.
10. Seeman E. Osteocytes—martyrs for integrity of bone strength. Osteoporos Int. 2006;17(10):1443–8.
11. Vaananen HK, Laitala-Leinonen T. Osteoclast lineage and function. Arch Biochem Biophys. 2008;473(2):132–8.
12. Ho AYY, Kung AWC. Determinants of peak bone mineral density and bone area in young women. J Bone Miner Metab. 2005;23(6):470–5.
13. Matkovic V, Jelic T, Wardlaw GM, Ilich JZ, Goel PK, Wright JK, Andon MB, Smith KT, Heaney RP. Timing of peak bone mass in Caucasian females and its implication for the prevention of osteoporosis. Inference from a cross-sectional model. J Clin Invest. 1994;93(2):799–808.
14. Fan F, Xue WQ, Wu BH, He MG, Xie HL, Ouyang WF, Tu SL, Chen YM. Higher fish intake is associated with a lower risk of hip fractures in Chinese men and women: a matched case-control study. PLoS One. 2013;8(2):e56849.
15. Zalloua PA, Hsu Y-H, Terwedow H, Zang T, Wu D, Tang G, Li Z, Hong X, Azar ST, Wang B, Bouxsein ML, Brain J, Cummings SR, Rosen CJ, Xu X. Impact of seafood and fruit consumption on bone mineral density. Maturitas. 2007;56(1):1–11.
16. Xu Z, Chen H, Fan FJ, Shi PJ, Tu ML, Cheng SZ, Wang ZY, Du M. Bone formation activity of an osteogenic dodecapeptide from blue mussels (*Mytilus edulis*). Food Funct. 2019;10(9):5616–25.
17. Xu Z, Chen H, Wang ZY, Fan FJ, Shi PJ, Tu ML, Du M. Isolation and characterization of peptides from Mytilus edulis with osteogenic activity in mouse MC3T3-E1 preosteoblast cells. J Agric Food Chem. 2019;67(5):1572–84.
18. Chen H, Xu Z, Fan FJ, Shi PJ, Tu ML, Wang ZY, Du M. Identification and mechanism evaluation of a novel osteogenesis promoting peptide from Tubulin alpha-1C chain in *Crassostrea gigas*. Food Chem. 2019;272:751–7.
19. Hyung JH, Ahn CB, Je JY. Blue mussel (*Mytilus edulis*) protein hydrolysate promotes mouse mesenchymal stem cell differentiation into osteoblasts through upregulation of bone morphogenetic protein. Food Chem. 2018;242:156–61.
20. Hyung JH, Ahn CB, Je JY. Osteoblastogenic activity of ark shell protein hydrolysates with low molecular weight in mouse mesenchymal stem cells. RSC Adv. 2016;6(35):29365–70.
21. Oh Y, Ahn CB, Hyung JH, Je JY. Two novel peptides from ark shell protein stimulate osteoblast differentiation and rescue ovariectomy-induced bone loss. Toxicol Appl Pharmacol. 2019;385:114779.
22. De Marco R, Tolomelli A, Juaristi E, Gentilucci L. Integrin ligands with α/β-hybrid peptide structure: design, bioactivity, and conformational aspects. Med Res Rev. 2016;36(3):389–424.
23. Finney AC, Stokes KY, Pattillo CB, Orr AW. Integrin signaling in atherosclerosis. Cell Mol Life Sci. 2017;74(12):2263–82.
24. Taubenberger AV, Woodruff MA, Bai HF, Muller DJ, Hutmacher DW. The effect of unlocking RGD-motifs in collagen I on pre-osteoblast adhesion and differentiation. Biomaterials. 2010;31(10):2827–35.

25. Kaneko K, Ito M, Naoe Y, Lacy-Hulbert A, Ikeda K. Integrin αv in the mechanical response of osteoblast lineage cells. Biochem Biophys Res Commun. 2014;447(2):352–7.
26. Weiss MJ, Ray K, Henthorn PS, Lamb B, Kadesch T, Harris H. Structure of the human liver/bone/kidney alkaline phosphatase gene. J Biol Chem. 1988;263(24):12002–10.
27. Garnero P, Delmas PD. Assessment of the serum levels of bone alkaline phosphatase with a new immunoradiometric assay in patients with metabolic bone disease. J Clin Endocrinol Metab. 1993;77(4):1046–53.
28. Hoang QQ, Sicheri F, Howard AJ, Yang DSC. Bone recognition mechanism of porcine osteocalcin from crystal structure. Nature. 2003;425(6961):977–80.
29. Garnero P, Grimaux M, Seguin P, Delmas PD. Characterization of immunoreactive forms of human osteocalcin generated *in vivo* and *in vitro*. J Bone Miner Res. 1994;9(2):255–64.
30. Halleen JM, Tiitinen SL, Ylipahkala H, Fagerlund KM, Vaananen HK. Tartrate-resistant acid phosphatase 5b (TRACP 5b) as a marker of bone resorption. Clin Lab. 2006;52(9–10):499–509.
31. Garnero P, Ferreras M, Karsdal MA, Nicamhlaoibh R, Risteli J, Borel O, Qvist P, Delmas PD, Foged NT, Delaisse JM. The type I collagen fragments ICTP and CTX reveal distinct enzymatic pathways of bone collagen degradation. J Bone Miner Res Off J Am Soc Bone Miner Res. 2003;18(5):859–67.
32. Liu HX, Tu ML, Cheng SZ, Xu Z, Xu XB, Du M. Anticoagulant decapeptide interacts with thrombin at the active site and exosite-I. J Agric Food Chem. 2020;68(1):176–84.
33. Li YR, Huang YN, Zhao B, Wu MF, Li TY, Zhang YL, Chen D, Yu M, Mo W. RGD-hirudin-based low molecular weight peptide prevents blood coagulation via subcutaneous injection. Acta Pharmacol Sin. 2020;41(6):753–62.
34. Li P, Wang L, Ding Y, Wu B, Shu C, Nie A, Li S, Shen B, Rao Z. Crystallization and preliminary X-ray diffraction analysis of FKBP12 complexed with a novel neurotrophic ligand. Protein Pept Lett. 2002;9(5):459–63.
35. Baron R, Rawadi G. Wnt signaling and the regulation of bone mass. Curr Osteoporos Rep. 2007;5(2):73–80.
36. Perugorria MJ, Olaizola P, Labiano I, Esparza-Baquer A, Marzioni M, Marin JJG, Bujanda L, Banales JM. Wnt-β-catenin signalling in liver development, health and disease. Nat Rev Gastroenterol Hepatol. 2019;16(2):121–36.
37. Pivonka P, Zimak J, Smith DW, Gardiner BS, Dunstan CR, Sims NA, Martin TJ, Mundy GR. Theoretical investigation of the role of the RANK-RANKL-OPG system in bone remodeling. J Theor Biol. 2010;262(2):306–16.
38. Vega D, Maalouf NM, Sakhaee K. CLINICAL review #: the role of receptor activator of nuclear factor-kappaB (RANK)/RANK ligand/osteoprotegerin: clinical implications. J Clin Endocrinol Metab. 2007;92(12):4514–21.
39. Horbelt D, Denkis A, Knaus P. A portrait of transforming growth factor β superfamily signalling: background matters. Int J Biochem Cell Biol. 2012;44(3):469–74.
40. Kopf J, Paarmann P, Hiepen C, Horbelt D, Knaus P. BMP growth factor signaling in a biomechanical context. Biofactors. 2014;40(2):171–87.
41. Layden MJ, Martindale MQ. Non-canonical Notch signaling represents an ancestral mechanism to regulate neural differentiation. EvoDevo. 2014;5:30.
42. Regan J, Long FX. Notch signaling and bone remodeling. Curr Osteoporos Rep. 2013;11(2):126–9.

Chapter 6
Marine Shellfish Peptides and Hypertension

Ming Du, Shuzhen Cheng, Peifan Li, and Baifeng Fu

Abstract This section explores the mechanisms behind hypertension. It also examines the potential of marine shellfish-derived peptides in managing hypertension. This is especially true for peptides with angiotensin-converting enzyme (ACE) inhibitory activity. ACE inhibitors play a crucial role in regulating blood pressure. They prevent angiotensin I from converting to angiotensin II. Angiotensin II is a peptide that causes vasoconstriction. Marine peptides from shellfish are being studied. These shellfish include oysters, mussels, and abalones. Researchers are looking at their ACE-inhibiting properties. They also study their potential to improve endothelial function. These peptides show promise as treatments for hypertension. Future research should focus on several areas. It should identify and optimize these peptides. It should also explore their preparation methods and bioactivity.

Keywords Hypertension · Angiotensin-converting enzyme inhibition · Marine shellfish peptides

Hypertension is a widespread chronic condition. It is characterized by elevated arterial blood pressure. It is also linked to severe cardiovascular, cerebrovascular, and renal diseases. These conditions significantly affect quality of life. Several factors contribute to hypertension. They include genetics, lifestyle, and dysfunction in various physiological systems of the body. Angiotensin-converting enzyme (ACE) converts angiotensin I to angiotensin II. Angiotensin II raises blood pressure by constricting blood vessels. Inhibiting ACE reduces the production of angiotensin II. This, in turn, lowers blood pressure. Marine organisms have complex and unique chemical structures in their secondary metabolites. They also have distinctive,

M. Du
College of Food Science and Engineering, Dalian Ocean University, Dalian, China

S. Cheng (✉)
School of Food Science and Technology, Dalian Polytechnic University, Dalian, China

P. Li · B. Fu
Food Science and Engineering, Dalian Polytechnic University, Dalian, China

M. Du, S. Cheng (eds.), *Bioactive Proteins and Peptides from Marine Shellfish*,
https://doi.org/10.1007/978-981-95-3937-6_6

potent bioactivities. For these reasons, they have become an important resource. They help in discovering innovative drugs and novel bioproducts. Marine shellfish-derived peptides lower blood pressure through multiple mechanisms. These include inhibiting ACE activity and improving vascular endothelial function. They show considerable therapeutic potential. This chapter provides an overview. It focuses on the potential of bioactive peptides from marine shellfish in preventing and managing hypertension. It covers peptide screening, identification, preparation, and the underlying bioactive mechanisms.

6.1 Hypertension and Angiotensin-Converting Enzyme

6.1.1 Factors Contributing to Hypertension

Hypertension is characterized by elevated systemic arterial blood pressure (systolic pressure ≥130 mm Hg and/or diastolic pressure ≥80 mm Hg) and is often associated with functional or organic damage to organs such as the heart, brain, and kidneys. The condition is generally asymptomatic, but when blood pressure reaches certain levels, it may lead to typical symptoms, such as dizziness, headaches, arrhythmias, palpitations, and tinnitus. Chronic hypertension is a major risk factor for stroke, coronary artery disease, heart failure, atrial fibrillation, peripheral artery disease, visual impairment, chronic kidney disease, and dementia.

Hypertension can be triggered by various factors. These include genetics, age, body weight, environmental factors, medication intake, and other health conditions. Clinically, hypertension is divided into two types. The first is essential (primary) hypertension, which has no identifiable cause. The second is secondary hypertension, which has a specific underlying cause. Primary hypertension makes up over 90% of all hypertension cases. It is an independent condition mainly characterized by elevated blood pressure. The exact mechanism of primary hypertension is not fully understood. However, extensive experimental research and clinical observations show that genetics plays a strong role in its development.

Recent studies have shown that patients with primary hypertension often have abnormalities in ion transport across cell membranes. This has a strong genetic link. However, more research is needed to find out if this is a causal mechanism in hypertension development. Unhealthy lifestyle factors increase the risk of hypertension. These include a high-sodium, low-potassium diet, lack of physical activity, excess body weight, smoking, and alcohol consumption. Body weight has a significant influence on blood pressure in children. Poor weight control during childhood can greatly raise the risk of hypertension in adulthood. Additionally, certain factors may contribute to elevated blood pressure. These include heightened sympathetic nervous activity, stress, and insufficient sleep. They can speed up the production of adrenaline and noradrenaline. But there is still no conclusive evidence that these factors directly cause hypertension. Arterial blood pressure is largely determined by two things: cardiac output and total peripheral resistance. Some factors can increase cardiac output. Examples include blood volume expansion from sodium and water retention, or increased myocardial contractility. Other factors can raise peripheral resistance, such as peripheral vasoconstriction influenced by neural or endocrine factors. Both types of factors can elevate blood pressure. Besides direct causes, some indirect factors can also contribute to hypertension. These include psychological stress and certain endocrine hormones. These indirect influences mainly affect blood pressure by acting on key regulatory systems. The renin–angiotensin–aldosterone system is particularly important in this process.

Hypertension caused by an identifiable underlying factor is called secondary hypertension. It accounts for about 5–10% of all hypertensive cases. Common causes include chronic kidney disease, renal artery stenosis, endocrine disorders, and the use of contraceptives. Kidney disorders, especially renovascular diseases, can have several effects. They can reduce renal perfusion pressure or effective circulating blood volume. They can also increase sympathetic nervous activity. All these factors stimulate juxtaglomerular cells to secrete large amounts of renin. Renin is a proteolytic enzyme. It catalyzes the hydrolysis of angiotensinogen into angiotensin I. Angiotensinogen is an α2-globulin produced by the liver, and angiotensin I is an inactive precursor. When angiotensin I flows through vascular beds, especially in the pulmonary circulation, it is converted by ACE into active angiotensin II. Angiotensin II is a powerful vasoconstrictor. It raises blood pressure directly. It also indirectly stimulates the zona glomerulosa of the adrenal cortex to secrete aldosterone. Aldosterone promotes sodium retention in the renal tubules. This expands blood volume and further increases blood pressure. Epinephrine raises systolic blood pressure. It does this by increasing cardiac output through stronger myocardial contractility and a faster heart rate. Norepinephrine has these effects too. Additionally, it strongly constricts peripheral vessels. This leads to higher levels of both systolic and diastolic blood pressure. In cases of aortic coarctation, the mechanical obstruction causes hypertension in the upper limbs. But in some advanced cases, blood pressure may stay high even after surgery to relieve the coarctation. This might be due to increased renin levels or higher peripheral vascular resistance. Renin plays a crucial role in the development of hypertension.

The occurrence of hypertension is closely related to various inducing factors. First, genetic factors play a role. Children of hypertensive parents have a 46% higher likelihood of developing hypertension. Second, smoking, especially heavy smoking, leads to arteriosclerosis. This condition increases blood pressure. Third, obesity is a major cause of elevated blood pressure. Fourth, excessive alcohol consumption is another known risk factor for hypertension. Finally, other contributing factors include the use of certain medications.

6.1.2 Role of ACE in the Pathogenesis of Hypertension

Angiotensin-converting enzyme (ACE) is a critical component of the renin–angiotensin system (RAS). This system regulates blood pressure by controlling the volume of blood in the vessels. ACE converts inactive angiotensin I into active angiotensin II. This conversion leads to vasoconstriction, which indirectly raises blood pressure. ACE inhibitors are commonly used to treat cardiovascular diseases. In 1956, Leonard first identified ACE [1], and in 2002, Natesh first determined the crystal structure of human testicular ACE, publishing the findings in *Nature* in January 2003 [2]. Besides being present in pulmonary capillaries, ACE is also expressed in endothelial and renal epithelial cells. In addition to activating angiotensin I, ACE is capable of degrading bradykinin [3], substance P, and amyloid β protein [4].

Angiotensin I is a peptide made up of 10 amino acids, with the sequence DRVYIHPFHL. It is generated from angiotensinogen under the action of renin. Through ACE, the C-terminal dipeptide (His-Leu) is removed. This process converts the inactive decapeptide angiotensin I (Ang I) into the biologically active octapeptide angiotensin II (Ang II). Ang II is an effective vasoconstrictor, and its action depends on substrate concentration. It binds to the angiotensin II type 1 receptor (AT1). This binding triggers a series of physiological responses. These responses lead to vasoconstriction and increased blood pressure [5]. In addition, ACE is also part of the kallikrein-kinin system. It can degrade bradykinin, a peptide with vasodilatory properties. It can also degrade other vasoactive peptides (Fig. 6.1).

ACE is a zinc metalloprotease. Zinc ions are crucial for its activity because they directly participate in the catalytic process of peptide bond hydrolysis. For this reason, ACE can be inhibited by metal chelators [7, 8]. In the catalytic mechanism of ACE, the glutamate residue (E384) has a dual function. On one hand, it acts as a general base, making water a nucleophilic agent. On the other hand, it functions as a general acid to assist in peptide bond cleavage [9]. Under physiological conditions, ACE exhibits approximately 60% of its maximal activity toward angiotensin I. It shows full activity toward bradykinin, however. Hence, the ion activation function of ACE is considered to be highly substrate-specific (Fig. 6.2).

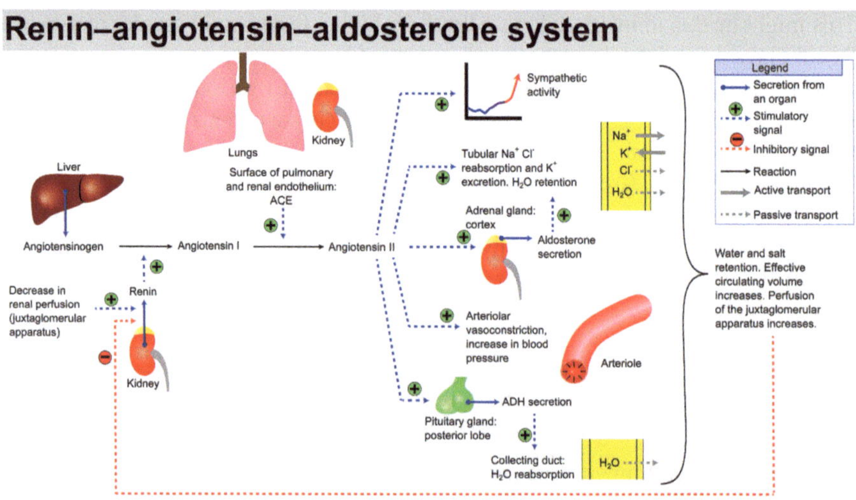

Fig. 6.1 Diagram of the renin–angiotensin system [6]

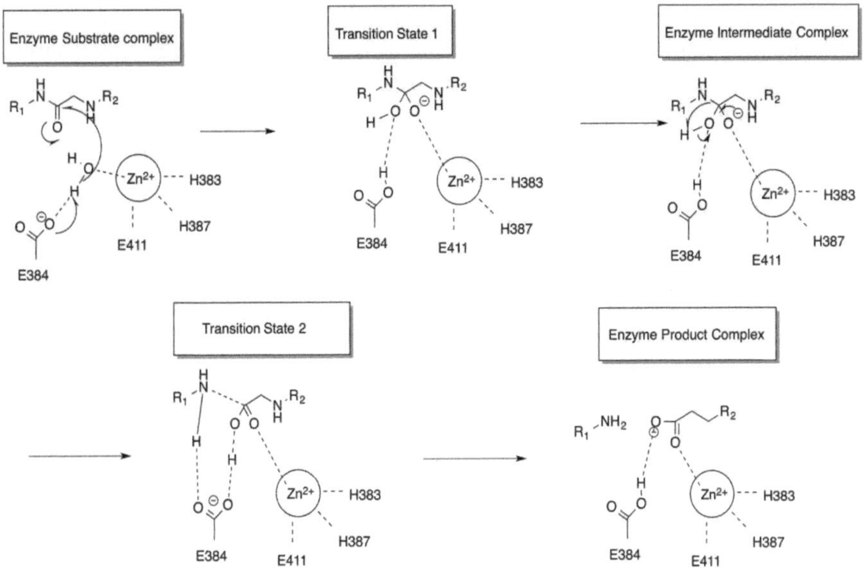

Fig. 6.2 The catalytic hydrolysis mechanism of ACE [10]

ACE inhibitors are a class of first-line drugs used to treat hypertension and heart failure. Their mechanism of action involves promoting vasodilation and reducing blood volume. This, in turn, lowers blood pressure. ACE inhibitors work by inhibiting the activity of angiotensin-converting enzyme. They reduce the enzyme's conversion of angiotensin I into angiotensin II. They also inhibit the hydrolysis of bradykinin. As a result, ACE inhibitors decrease the production of angiotensin II, a vasoconstrictor. At the same time, they increase the levels of bradykinin, a vasodilatory peptide. This creates a synergistic effect in lowering blood pressure. Currently, commonly prescribed ACE inhibitors in clinical practice include benazepril, zofenopril, perindopril, captopril, enalapril, lisinopril, and ramipril.

6.2 Preparation and Identification of ACE Inhibitory Peptides

6.2.1 ACE Inhibitory Peptides

With the growing emphasis on nutrition and health, the development of food-derived ACE inhibitory peptides has become a prominent research area. In recent years, significant progress has been made in extracting bioactive peptides with ACE inhibitory activity from food-derived proteins. These proteins come from a wide variety of food sources. They include common ingredients such as meat, eggs, dairy, fruits, vegetables, and seafood.

The ocean covers 70% of the Earth's surface. Therefore, the development and utilization of marine resources are crucial to human progress. Marine organisms have adapted to extreme environments over the long term. These environments include high salinity, extreme temperatures, high pressure, and limited nutrient availability. As a result, their protein structures and amino acid sequences are distinct from those of terrestrial organisms. This unique feature makes marine proteins a valuable resource for identifying novel ACE inhibitory peptides. Commonly consumed shellfish include oysters, mussels, scallops, clams, abalones, and sea snails. A review of relevant literature shows that ACE inhibitory peptides from oysters and mussels have been more extensively studied. In contrast, research on ACE inhibitory peptides from other shellfish sources is relatively limited. Therefore, future research should focus on exploring additional shellfish sources to identify more potent ACE inhibitory peptides (Table 6.1).

6.2.2 Preparation and Identification of ACE Inhibitory Peptides

The classical methods for extracting bioactive peptides from food sources typically include the following steps. First, select and prepare protein sources. Then, choose proteases or microorganisms. Next, perform protein hydrolysis or fermentation. After that, separate bioactive components based on specific activities. Use various separation techniques, such as desalting, ultrafiltration, ethanol precipitation, and chromatography. Identify bioactive peptide sequences using MS/MS. Synthesize the bioactive peptides. Finally, validate the activity of the homogenized peptides.

With the continuous development of bioinformatics, researchers have been developing new preparation methods. For example, methods based on qualitative structure–activity relationships combined with bioinformatics have been developed. These methods predict bioactive peptides in food protein sources [32]. With the isolation and purification of a large number of bioactive peptides, various quantitative structure-activity relationship (QSAR) models have been developed to predict their applicability for different therapeutic purposes. As different modeling approaches (through the application of various descriptors) increase, selecting the appropriate method to save time and costs has become crucial.

When constructing QSAR models, the data selected are crucial to the effectiveness of the model. A review of published studies shows that most rely on literature or databases to obtain the necessary data. Currently, commonly used databases in QSAR model construction include ACEpepDB, BIOPEP, EROP Moscow, PepBank, and PeptideDB. These databases provide bioactive peptides with verified efficacy. These peptides consist of 2–14 amino acids and are valuable resources for QSAR model construction. Regarding modeling methods, linear regression models and nonlinear models are the most commonly used techniques. Linear regression models include multiple linear regression, ordinary least squares, principal component

Table 6.1 ACE inhibitory peptides from marine shellfish sources

Peptide sequence (mixture)	IC50/ACE	Preparation	Study of the mechanism of activity	Source
EVMAGNLYPG	1.01 mg/mL	Fermentation	Spontaneously hypertensive rats (SHR)	Blue mussel [11]
VISDEDGVTH	8.16 μM	Fermentation	Human umbilical vein endothelial cells (HUVECs), SHR	*Ruditapes philippinarum* [12]
YN	51 μM	Enzymatic hydrolysis (complex protease)		Hard clam [13]
ATPGDEG	0.39 mg/mL	Boiling	SHR	Abalone [14]
AMN	106.24 μg/mL	Enzymatic hydrolysis (alkaline protease—papain)		Abalone [15]
DLTDY	143 μM	Enzymatic hydrolysis (trypsin)	SHR	Oyster [16]
VQY	9.8 μM	Enzymatic hydrolysis (pepsin, trypsin, alkaline enzymes, flavor enzymes)		Razor Clam [17]
SAP, AMP, TSGP	0.032 mg/mL	Enzymatic hydrolysis (chymosin and proline-specific endopeptidase)		Oyster [18]
LF	126 μM	Enzymatic hydrolysis (deoxyribonuclease)		Oyster [19]
GVGSPY	5.82 μg/mL	Enzymatic hydrolysis		Pearl oyster [20]
HLHT, GWA	458.06 μM, 109.25 μM	Enzymatic hydrolysis (alkaline protease)		Pearl oyster [21]
GRVSNCAA TYLPVH	57.93 μM 1.37 μM		HUVECs Hepatocytes SHR	*Ruditapes philippinarum* [22]
IAE, IVE, FE, ALAFE, VEV, AEL, LVE, PLG	34.7 μM, 95.6 μM, 51.8 μM, 167.5 μM, 8.7 μM, 57.1 μM, 14.2 μM, 72.1 μM	Enzymatic hydrolysis (pepsin)	SHR	*Ruditapes philippinarum*, Pearl oyster [23]
Mixture	0.3 mg/mL	Enzymatic hydrolysis (trypsin and chymotrypsin)		Oyster [24]
Mixture	3.34 μg/mL	Thermal processing		Oyster [25]

(continued)

Table 6.1 (continued)

Peptide sequence (mixture)	IC50/ACE	Preparation	Study of the mechanism of activity	Source
Mixture	78.18% (2 mg/mL)	Enzymatic hydrolysis (pepsin, bromelain, and papain)		Oyster [26]
Mixture	88.1% (unspecified)	Subcritical water extraction		Blue mussel [27]
Mixture	2.45 mg/mL, 0.0874 mg/mL	Fermentation	SHR	Oyster [28]
Mixture	1.13–3.34 mg/mL	Enzymatic hydrolysis (alkaline protease)		Blue mussel [29]
Mixture	20–25% (34.64 μg/mL)	Enzymatic hydrolysis (alkaline protease)		Blue mussel [30]
Mixture	90.28% (50 mg/mL)	pressurized hot water extraction		Oyster [31]

regression, and partial least squares. Nonlinear models include artificial neural networks. In recent years, support vector machines have also been frequently applied in model construction. QSAR analysis is typically based on linear models. These models use molecular descriptors as linear functions to predict biological activity. Particularly when the descriptors are optimized for specific biological activities, linear models can effectively analyze and predict data for similar small molecule compounds with high accuracy.

He et al. constructed a QSAR model for ACE inhibitory peptides using artificial neural networks based on the structural or activity data of 58 ACE inhibitory peptides [33]. The results indicated that the C-terminal of the peptide chain plays a crucial role in the bioactivity of ACE inhibitory peptides. Specifically, peptides with hydrophobic amino acids at the C-terminus exhibited stronger ACE inhibitory activity. Proteins rich in hydrophobic amino acids are also more likely to yield highly effective ACE inhibitory peptides. Additionally, the established QSAR model revealed that alkaline protease is the optimal enzyme for generating ACE inhibitory peptides. Beyond assisting in the selection of suitable enzymes, QSAR methods also play an important role in screening potential food source proteins for ACE inhibitory peptide preparation. Yuchen Gu et al. used a QSAR-assisted computer simulation method. They simulated the digestion of proteins from 15 common foods with thermophilic protease. This process generated 5709 peptides, each composed of 2–6 amino acid residues. Based on predicted bioactivity, the peptides were classified into three categories. Proteins from pork, beef, and chicken contained the highest levels of effective peptides (IC50 < 10 μM). They were followed by proteins from milk, eggs, soybeans, and canola oil. In contrast, proteins from fish (excluding salmon) and grains (oats and barley) had the lowest levels of effective peptides. This study indicates that proteins from livestock, poultry, milk, eggs, soybeans, and canola oil are good sources of ACE inhibitory peptides [32]. In applying QSAR methods to screen for ACE inhibitory peptides, certain physicochemical properties are often used as the primary "descriptive language" of peptides. These include hydrophobicity, charge, spatial conformation, and hydrogen bond interactions. Shu developed a novel QSAR method successfully. This was done by introducing size as an additional physicochemical property and using the least squares method [34]. Compared to traditional approaches, this method demonstrated superior predictive results for ACE inhibitory peptide activity.

The use of QSAR methods to screen for ACE precursor proteins and biocatalytic enzymes helps save time. After selecting the appropriate ACE precursor proteins and enzymes, ACE affinity chromatography is used to separate and purify the enzymatic hydrolysates. This method not only simplifies traditional, complex purification processes but also further reduces time and costs. In the affinity chromatography purification process, preparing a column with immobilized ACE enzyme is a critical step. It directly impacts purification efficiency and precision. Therefore, careful research is required when selecting an appropriate ACE enzyme for immobilization. Feng et al. used ACE extract from pig lungs and immobilized it on a novel substrate, magnetite (Fe_3O_4), to develop an innovative ACE chromatography column for purifying ACE inhibitory peptides from the enzymatic hydrolysate of wakame [35].

Rapid determination of ACE activity is essential for the preparation and screening of ACE inhibitory peptides, significantly reducing time and costs. He et al. used capillary electrophoresis to quickly measure the IC50 values of ACE inhibitory peptides in hydrolysates from 48 marine proteins [36]. Siemerink employed rapid liquid chromatography/mass spectrometry (LC/MS) screening techniques to efficiently identify ACE inhibitors from complex natural mixtures such as snake venom [37]. Migue developed a rapid method for detecting ACE enzyme activity. This was achieved by substituting the ACE enzyme substrate. The method simplified the traditional two-step detection process into a single-step method. This advancement greatly improved detection efficiency. It also reduced the error rate in ACE activity assays [38].

6.3 Mechanisms of Bioactive Peptides

Angiotensin-converting enzyme (ACE, EC 3.4.15.1) is a dipeptidyl carboxypeptidase containing two highly similar protein domains (N- and C-domains), each with a zinc ion-containing catalytic center [39, 40]. The ACE gene in mammals originated through gene duplication during vertebrate evolution. Studies using domain-selective inhibitors and ACE gene knockout mice have revealed that the C-terminal domain of mammalian ACE is the primary region responsible for cleaving Ang I to Ang II [39, 41]. In addition, both the N-terminal and C-terminal domains of ACE participate in the inactivation of bradykinin in the bloodstream. Each domain contributes similarly to this process. In a single free-state system, both the N-terminal and C-terminal domains are essential [42]. Another important physiological substrate of ACE is Ac-SDKP, which acts as a regulator of hematopoietic stem cell and fibroblast proliferation and is involved in the regulation of vascular remodeling and inflammation. Its degradation is entirely controlled by the N-terminal domain of ACE [43]. A reduction in Ac-SDKP levels may lead to increased blood pressure. It may also raise the risk of cardiovascular diseases. Therefore, ACE is an important drug target for treating cardiovascular diseases. Its metabolic effects on Ang II and bradykinin in the circulation form the physiological basis for the blood pressure-lowering effects of ACE inhibitors. Current ACE inhibitors generally lack domain specificity. This limitation leads to elevated bradykinin levels in the body. The accumulation of bradykinin is a well-known trigger for adverse reactions. These include cough and angioedema. While C-terminal domain-selective ACE inhibitors may lower blood pressure by reducing Ang II, they may also increase the risk of side effects in patients. High-resolution crystal structure analysis has revealed significant differences. These differences exist between the N-terminal and C-terminal domains of ACE in the framework of the active site. This helps explain why the two domains exhibit different selectivity and activity toward specific substrates.

The first ACE inhibitory peptides displaying antihypertensive properties were members of the natural bradykinin-potentiating peptide family. They are derived from snake venom. Interestingly, some of these bradykinins exhibit selectivity for the C-terminal domain of ACE. They are characterized by an N-terminal pyroglutamic acid residue and a C-terminal Pro-Pro dipeptide. These features result in strong competitive inhibition of Ang I cleavage. The ACE inhibitors currently used in clinical practice all contain an ionizable group. This group coordinates with the zinc at the active site. This indicates their inhibitory mechanisms differ from those of natural peptide inhibitors. Although several crystal structures of ACE inhibitor complexes have been determined in recent years, structural data on natural peptide complexes remain relatively scarce.

6.3.1 Biochemical Methods

The ACE inhibitory capacity of bioactive peptides is typically expressed as the IC50 value. This value represents the concentration of the inhibitor. It is the concentration required to inhibit 50% of ACE activity. The IC50 value is a key indicator. It reflects the bioactivity potency of peptide compounds. It is also crucial for screening and evaluating potential antihypertensive peptides. The measurement of ACE inhibitory activity typically involves three methods. These methods are spectrophotometric, fluorometric, and high-performance liquid chromatography (HPLC). These methods assess ACE activity and inhibition. They do this by monitoring changes in absorbance, fluorescence intensity, or chromatographic peaks. The substrates used in in vitro assays differ from ACE's natural substrates. The natural substrates are Ang I or bradykinin. However, these synthetic peptide analogs remain effective. They are effective in characterizing ACE inhibitory activity.

1. Lineweaver–Burk Method

   Sheih determined the Km and Vmax of ACE inhibitory peptides and used the Lineweaver–Burk method. This method established that these peptides bind to ACE in a noncompetitive manner to exert an inhibitory effect [44]. Wang used the same method to confirm that ACE inhibitory peptides derived from oysters also act as noncompetitive inhibitors [45].
2. Molecular Docking Method

   Pan et al. utilized flexible molecular docking techniques to investigate the molecular mechanisms, binding sites, types, and energies of the interaction between Leu-Leu and ACE [46]. Li et al. explored the binding mechanisms at the molecular level through docking experiments, identifying that the seven residues in the active site of ACE (His383, His387, Glu384, Arg522, Asp358, Ala356, and Asn70) have strong interactions with two atoms (O5 and H60) of ACHEP, which play a crucial role in the stability of the binding [47]. Xue et al. employed molecular docking technology. They studied the potential key targets and mechanisms of the ACE inhibitory peptide Asn-Cys-Trp (NCW). They identified 11 potential key antihypertensive targets. They found that peptide NCW has a high affinity for these targets. Hydrogen bonds are the primary interaction force between NCW and the targets [48].
3. Isothermal Titration Calorimetry

   Ni used isothermal titration calorimetry. Ni explored the inhibitory mode of the yeast-derived bioactive peptide TPTQQS on ACE. The study demonstrated that this peptide binds to ACE in a noncompetitive manner. This binding inhibits ACE's conversion of angiotensin I. The Lineweaver–Burk method was also employed. It further confirmed that this peptide acts as a noncompetitive inhibitor [49].

6.3.2 Cellular Model

In cellular models, a primary approach involves the use of a free radical protection model. Himaya examined several markers. These include lipid and protein oxidation markers, intracellular reactive oxygen species (ROS) levels, and the gene expression of intracellular antioxidant enzymes. The antioxidant enzymes are superoxide dismutase, glutathione, and catalase. The examination was conducted in human lung fibroblasts and mouse monocytes. The study found that ACE inhibitory peptides effectively scavenge intracellular ROS. They do this by upregulating the mRNA expression of cellular antioxidant enzymes. This action significantly reduces oxidation levels. The reduced oxidation levels involve membrane lipids, proteins, and DNA in RAW264.7 cells. This process protects cells from ROS-mediated damage [50].

6.3.3 *Animal Model*

1. Spontaneously Hypertensive Rat Model

   The spontaneously hypertensive rat (SHR) model was developed by breeding male Wistar Kyoto rats with higher systolic blood pressure (150–175 mm Hg) with female Wistar Kyoto rats with relatively lower systolic blood pressure (130–140 mm Hg). All offspring with systolic blood pressure over 150 mm Hg were selected, followed by inbreeding among high blood pressure offspring. After 20 generations of selective inbreeding, a stable SHR strain with hereditary high blood pressure was established.
2. Renal Hypertension Rat Model

   Zhao created the two-kidney, one-clip (2K1C) hypertension model. This was done by inserting a 0.4 mm silver clip on the left renal artery. The model simulates hypertension symptoms. These symptoms are caused by renal issues in humans. After 1 month of oral gavage, blood pressure was measured. Carotid cannulation was used for the measurement. The results showed that oral administration of ACE inhibitory peptides significantly reduced systolic and diastolic blood pressure. This reduction occurred in the renal hypertensive rats. The findings suggest the antihypertensive effect of ACE inhibitory peptides through oral intake [51].
3. Isolated Artery

   "Isolated artery" refers to an artery. It has been removed from the organism for experimental study. To explore the antihypertensive mechanism of ACE inhibitory peptides in vascular tissue, functional evidence in vascular tissue is necessary. This can be achieved through in vitro testing on isolated arteries. ACE in the arterial wall can locally form Ang I. This process is essential for inducing vasoconstriction [52, 53].
4. In Vivo ACE Activity Measurement

   ACE is a key component. It helps maintain normal blood pressure and electrolyte balance. It is also central to the renin–angiotensin system (RAS). Its primary function is to cleave Ang I into Ang II. It also degrades bradykinin. The in vivo inhibition of ACE can be evaluated through two methods. One method is measuring the activity of tissue-bound or circulating soluble ACE. The other is assessing the levels of Ang II in circulation [54].

6.4 Other Targets for Hypertension Treatment

A new direction in hypertension treatment involves regulating the RAS. This is done by inhibiting the AT1 receptor. Angiotensin receptor blockers, such as valsartan, can achieve this effect. These drugs bind to the AT1 receptor. This binding inhibits vasoconstriction and other cellular effects of Ang II. In vitro functional assays can be used. These assays use isolated arteries. They help evaluate the inhibitory effects of active peptides. The effects are on Ang II-induced, AT1 receptor-mediated vasoconstriction [55, 56].

The endothelin system is also a primary target for antihypertensive drug therapy. Blood pressure can be reduced by two approaches. One is inhibiting endothelin-converting enzyme (ECE). The other is antagonizing endothelin receptor systems. Selective ECE inhibitors have been tested. They were tested in hypertensive rat models. ECE receptor antagonists have been approved. They are approved for the treatment of pulmonary hypertension. They are also under clinical development. This development is for the treatment of systemic hypertension.

Currently, high-throughput technologies provide robust support. They help understand the molecular basis of bioactive compounds. Antihypertensive peptide molecules target multiple pathways. High-throughput methods are an effective strategy. They are used for identifying new targets. DNA microarray technology was used. It analyzed gene expression changes in the aorta of SHR. The analysis was done after repeated administration of casein-derived Val-Pro-Pro (VPP) and Ile-Pro-Pro (IPP). Significant differences were observed. These differences were in the expression of genes related to vascular function. Examples include endothelial nitric oxide synthase (eNOS), gap junction protein 40 (GJ40), and nuclear factor kappa B (NF-κB) genes. In the arachidonic acid pathway, treatment with VPP and IPP caused a slight increase. This increase was in cyclooxygenase (COX-1) expression. Meanwhile, peroxisome proliferator-activated receptor gamma (PPARγ) showed a significant reduction. PPARγ is a gene related to cytokine production [57]. This technology has also been used. It studies the molecular mechanisms of the antihypertensive effects of fermented milk. Differential gene expression is associated with hypertension. This expression occurs in the left ventricle of SHR. It relates to several processes. These include NO synthesis, cell proliferation, endothelin binding, and thrombolysis. The regulation of certain genes may represent key mechanisms. These genes include eNOS, PPARγ, and endothelin type A receptor. These mechanisms allow fermented milk to exert its potential antihypertensive effects [58].

6.5 Summary

In recent years, significant progress has been made. This progress is in the study of food-derived antihypertensive peptides. However, several aspects still require further development. These aspects include the production, characterization, and activity measurement of these peptides. Current research primarily involves using computational methods. These methods are used to virtually hydrolyze proteins. Researchers then synthesize peptides from these virtual hydrolysis predictions. They also verify the activity of these peptides. If the in vitro activity is confirmed, actual enzymatic hydrolysis is performed. The in vitro activity typically targets renin and angiotensin-converting enzyme. The hydrolysis is done to obtain peptides. This is followed by further in vitro and in vivo testing. Additionally, more clinical trials are needed. They will provide solid efficacy data. This data would enable foods or supplements containing antihypertensive peptides. They could then legally claim health benefits.

References

1. Skeggs LT, Kahn JR, Shumway NP. The preparation and function of the hypertensin-converting enzyme. J Exp Med. 1956;103(3):295–9.
2. Natesh R, Schwager SLU, Sturrock ED, Acharya KR. Crystal structure of the human angiotensin-converting enzyme–lisinopril complex. Nature. 2003;421(6922):551–4.
3. Filardi P. ACEi and ARBS in hypertension and heart failure. Cham: Springer International Publishing; 2015.
4. Hemming ML, Selkoe DJ. Amyloid β-protein is degraded by cellular angiotensin-converting enzyme (ACE) and elevated by an ACE inhibitor. J Biol Chem. 2005;280(45):37644–50.
5. Zhang R, Xu X, Chen T, Li L, Rao P. An assay for angiotensin-converting enzyme using capillary zone electrophoresis. Anal Biochem. 2000;280(2):286–90.
6. Britannica, The Editors of Encyclopaedia. Renin-angiotensin system. Encyclopedia Britannica. 2024. Accessed 11 Nov 2024.
7. Bünning P. The functional role of zinc in angiotensin converting enzyme: implications for the enzyme mechanism. J Inorg Biochem. 1985;24(3):183–98.
8. Wang W, McKinnie SMK, Farhan M, Paul M, McDonald T, McLean B, Llorens-Cortes C, Hazra S, Murray AG, Vederas JC, Oudit GY. Angiotensin-converting enzyme 2 metabolizes and partially inactivates Pyr-Apelin-13 and Apelin-17. Hypertension. 2016;68(2):365–77.
9. Zhang C, Wu S, Xu D. Catalytic mechanism of angiotensin-converting enzyme and effects of the chloride ion. J Phys Chem B. 2013;117(22):6635–45.
10. Wikimedia Commons. File: ACE mechanism.png — Wikimedia Commons, the free media repository. 2023. Accessed 11 Nov 2024.
11. Je J-Y, Park P-J, Byun H-G, Jung W-K, Kim S-K. Angiotensin I converting enzyme (ACE) inhibitory peptide derived from the sauce of fermented blue mussel. Bioresour Technol. 2005;96(14):1624–9.
12. Chen Y, Gao X, Wei Y, Liu Q, Jiang Y, Zhao L, Ulaah S. Isolation, purification and the anti-hypertensive effect of a novel angiotensin I-converting enzyme (ACE) inhibitory peptide from *Ruditapes Philippinarum* fermented with *Bacillus Natto*. Food Funct. 2018;9(10):5230–7.
13. Tsai J-S, Chen J-L, Pan BS. ACE-inhibitory peptides identified from the muscle protein hydrolysate of hard clam (*Meretrix Lusoria*). Process Biochem. 2008;43(7):743–7.
14. Qian Z-J, Zhang YY, Oh G-W, Heo S-Y, Park WS, Choi I-W, Jung W-K. Antioxidant and angiotensin I converting enzyme inhibition effects and antihypertensive effect in spontaneously hypertensive rats of peptide isolated from boiled abalone by-products, *Hallotis Discus Hannai*. J Aquat Food Prod Technol. 2018;27(9):946–60.
15. Wu Q, Cai QF, Tao ZP, Sun LC, Shen JD, Zhang LJ, Liu G-M, Cao MJ. Purification and characterization of a novel angiotensin I-converting enzyme inhibitory peptide derived from abalone (*Haliotis Discus Hannai Ino*) gonads. Eur Food Res Technol. 2014;240(1):137–45.
16. Shiozaki K, Shiozaki M, Masuda J, Yamauchi A, Ohwada S, Nakano T, Yamaguchi T, Saito T, Muramoto K, Sato M. Identification of oyster-derived hypotensive peptide acting as angiotensin-I-converting enzyme inhibitor. Fish Sci. 2010;76(5):865–72.
17. Li Y, Sadiq FA, Fu L, Zhu H, Zhong M, Sohail M. Identification of angiotensin I-converting enzyme inhibitory peptides derived from enzymatic hydrolysates of razor clam *Sinonovacula Constricta*. Mar Drugs. 2016;14(6):110.
18. Zhang T, Li M, Fu X, Mou H. Purification and characterization of angiotensin I-converting enzyme (ACE) inhibitory peptides with specific structure X-Pro. Eur Food Res Technol. 2019;245(8):1743–53.
19. Matsumoto K, Ogikubo A, Yoshino T, Matsui T, Osajima Y. Separation and purification of angiotensin I converting enzyme inhibitory peptide in peptic hydrolyzate of oyster. J Food Sci Technol. 1994;41(9):589–94.

20. Sasaki C, Tamura S, Tohse R, Fujita S, Kikuchi M, Asada C, Nakamura Y. Isolation and identification of an angiotensin I-converting enzyme inhibitory peptide from pearl oyster (*Pinctada Fucata*) shell protein hydrolysate. Process Biochem. 2019;77:137–42.
21. Liu P, Lan X, Yaseen M, Wu S, Feng X, Zhou L, Sun J, Liao A, Liao D, Sun L. Purification, characterization and evaluation of inhibitory mechanism of ACE inhibitory peptides from pearl oyster (*Pinctada Fucata Martensii*) meat protein hydrolysate. Mar Drugs. 2019;17(8):463.
22. Zhang Y, Pan D, Yang Z, Gao X, Dang Y. Angiotensin I-converting enzyme (ACE) inhibitory and dipeptidyl peptidase-4 (DPP-IV) inhibitory activity of umami peptides from *Ruditapes Philippinarum*. LWT. 2021;144:111265.
23. Suetsuna K. Identification of antihypertensive peptides from peptic digest of the short-necked clam *Tapes Philippinarum* and the pearl oyster *Pinctada Fucata Martensii*. Fish Sci. 2002;68(1):233–5.
24. Tamari M, Kanda H. Inhibition of angiotensin 1-converting enzyme by phosphopeptides in proteolitic hydrolysates derived from oyster, *Crassostrea Gigas*. Bull Fac Educ Nagasaki Univ, Nat Sci 1999;61:41–51.
25. Guo Z, Zhao F, Chen H, Tu M, Tao S, Wang Z, Wu C, He S, Du M. Heat treatments of peptides from oyster (*Crassostrea Gigas*) and the impact on their digestibility and angiotensin I converting enzyme inhibitory activity. Food Sci Biotechnol. 2020;29(7):961–7.
26. Gomez HLR, Peralta JP, Tejano LA, Chang Y-W. In silico and *in vitro* assessment of Portuguese oyster (*Crassostrea Angulata*) proteins as precursor of bioactive peptides. Int J Mol Sci. 2019;20(20):5191.
27. Han JK, Sung SC, Jo MJ, Lee SC. Antioxidant, ACE inhibitory, and acetylcholinesterase inhibitory activities of subcritical water extract of blue mussel. Food Sci Biotechnol. 2018;27(3):847–51.
28. Je JY, Park JY, Jung W, Park PJ, Kim SK. Isolation of angiotensin I converting enzyme (ACE) inhibitor from fermented oyster sauce, *Crassostrea Gigas*. Food Chem. 2005; 93(1):25–9.
29. Neves AC, Harnedy PA, FitzGerald RJ. Angiotensin converting enzyme and dipeptidyl peptidase-IV inhibitory, and antioxidant activities of a blue mussel (*Mytilus edulis*) meat protein extract and its hydrolysates. J Aquat Food Prod Technol. 2016;25(8):1221–33.
30. Dai ZY, Zhang YP, Zhang H, Lu YB. Preparation and characterization of *Mytilus edulis* protein hydrolysates with ACE inhibitory activity. J Food Biochem. 2010;36(1):66–74.
31. Lee HJ, Saravana PS, Cho YN, Haq M, Chun BS. Extraction of bioactive compounds from oyster (*Crassostrea gigas*) by pressurized hot water extraction. J Supercrit Fluids. 2018;141:120–7.
32. Gu Y, Majumder K, Wu J. QSAR-aided in silico approach in evaluation of food proteins as precursors of ACE inhibitory peptides. Food Res Int. 2011;44(8):2465–74.
33. He R, Ma H, Zhao W, Qu W, Zhao J, Luo L, Zhu W. Modeling the QSAR of ACE-inhibitory peptides with ANN and its applied illustration. Int J Pept. 2012;2012:1–9.
34. Shu M, Cheng X, Zhang Y, Wang Y, Lin Y, Wang L, Lin Z. Predicting the activity of ACE inhibitory peptides with a novel mode of pseudo amino acid composition. Protein Pept Lett. 2011;18(12):1233–43.
35. Megías C, Pedroche J, del Mar Yust M, Alaiz M, Girón-Calle J, Millán F, Vioque J. Affinity purification of angiotensin converting enzyme inhibitory peptides using immobilized ACE. J Agric Food Chem. 2006;54(19):7120–4.
36. He H, Chen X, Wu H, Sun C, Zhang Y, Zhou B. High throughput and rapid screening of marine protein hydrolysates enriched in peptides with angiotensin-I-converting enzyme inhibitory activity by capillary electrophoresis. Bioresour Technol. 2007;98(18):3499–505.

37. Siemerink M, Schebb NH, Liesener A, Perchuc A, Schöni R, Wilmer M, Hayen H, Karst U, Vogel M. Development of a fast liquid chromatography/mass spectrometry screening method for angiotensin-converting enzyme (ACE) inhibitors in complex natural mixtures like snake venom. Rapid Comm Mass Spectrom. 2010;24(5):687–97.
38. Sentandreu M, Toldrá F. A rapid, simple and sensitive fluorescence method for the assay of angiotensin-I converting enzyme. Food Chem. 2006;97(3):546–54.
39. Watermeyer J, Kroger W, Sturrock E, Ehlers M. Angiotensin-converting enzyme – new insights into structure, biological significance and prospects for domain-selective inhibitors. Curr Enzyme Inhib. 2009;5(3):134–47.
40. Acharya KR, Sturrock ED, Riordan JF, Ehlers MRW. ACE revisited: a new target for structure-based drug design. Nat Rev Drug Discov. 2003;2(11):891–902.
41. van Esch JHM, Tom B, Dive V, Batenburg WW, Georgiadis D, Yiotakis A, van Gool JMG, de Bruijn RJA, de Vries R, Danser AHJ. Selective angiotensin-converting enzyme C-domain inhibition is sufficient to prevent angiotensin I–induced vasoconstriction. Hypertension. 2005;45(1):120–5.
42. Liu C, Liu J, Wang M, Zhang B, Wang E, Liu B, Zhang T. Construction and application of membrane-bound angiotensin-I converting enzyme system: a new approach for the evaluation of angiotensin-I converting enzyme inhibitory peptides. J Agric Food Chem. 2020;68(20):5723–31.
43. Rousseau A, Michaud A, Chauvet M-T, Lenfant M, Corvol P. The hemoregulatory peptide N-Acetyl-Ser-Asp-Lys-Pro is a natural and specific substrate of the N-terminal active site of human angiotensin-converting enzyme. J Biol Chem. 1995;270(8):3656–61.
44. Sheih I-C, Fang TJ, Wu T-K. Isolation and characterisation of a novel angiotensin I-converting enzyme (ACE) inhibitory peptide from the algae protein waste. Food Chem. 2009;115(1):279–84.
45. Wang J, Hu J, Cui J, Bai X, Du Y, Miyaguchi Y, Lin B. Purification and identification of a ACE inhibitory peptide from oyster proteins hydrolysate and the antihypertensive effect of hydrolysate in spontaneously hypertensive rats. Food Chem. 2008;111(2):302–8.
46. Pan D, Cao J, Guo H, Zhao B. Studies on purification and the molecular mechanism of a novel ACE inhibitory peptide from whey protein hydrolysate. Food Chem. 2012;130(1):121–6.
47. Li P, Jia J, Fang M, Zhang L, Guo M, Xie J, Xia Y, Zhou L, Wei D. *In vitro* and *in vivo* ACE inhibitory of pistachio hydrolysates and in silico mechanism of identified peptide binding with ACE. Process Biochem. 2014;49(5):898–904.
48. Xue W, Zhao W, Wu S, Yu Z. Potential key targets and mechanism of the Mizuhopecten yessoensis derived ACE inhibitory peptide Asn-Cys-Trp (NCW) via network pharmacology and molecular docking. Food Sci Anim Prod. 2023;1(4):9240041.
49. Ni H, Li L, Liu G, Hu S-Q. Inhibition mechanism and model of an angiotensin I-converting enzyme (ACE)-inhibitory hexapeptide from yeast (Saccharomyces cerevisiae). PLoS One. 2012;7(5):e37077.
50. Himaya SWA, Ngo D-H, Ryu B, Kim S-K. An active peptide purified from gastrointestinal enzyme hydrolysate of pacific cod skin gelatin attenuates angiotensin-1 converting enzyme (ACE) activity and cellular oxidative stress. Food Chem. 2012;132(4):1872–82.
51. Zhao Y, Li B, Liu Z, Dong S, Zhao X, Zeng M. Antihypertensive effect and purification of an ACE inhibitory peptide from sea cucumber gelatin hydrolysate. Process Biochem. 2007;42(12):1586–91.
52. Whalley ET, Amure YO, Lye RH. Analysis of the mechanism of action of bradykinin on human basilar artery *in vitro*. Naunyn Schmiedeberg's Arch Pharmacol. 1987;335(4):433–7.
53. Eglème C, Cressier F, Wood JM. Local formation of angiotensin II in the rat aorta: effect of endothelium. Br J Pharmacol. 1990;100(2):237–40.
54. Coates D. The angiotensin converting enzyme (ACE). Int J Biochem Cell Biol. 2003;35(6):769–73.

55. Taylor AA, Siragy H, Nesbitt S. Angiotensin receptor blockers: pharmacology, efficacy, and safety. J Clin Hypertens. 2011;13(9):677–86.
56. Sica DA. Angiotensin receptor blockers: new considerations in their mechanism of action. J Clin Hypertens. 2006;8(5):381–5.
57. Yamaguchi N, Kawaguchi K, Yamamoto N. Study of the mechanism of antihypertensive peptides VPP and IPP in spontaneously hypertensive rats by DNA microarray analysis. Eur J Pharmacol. 2009;620(1–3):71–7.
58. Chen Y, Zhong Z, Xue J, Yang J, Zhang Q, Yue J, Zhang H. DNA microarray analysis of the antihypertensive effect of milk fermented by Lactobacillus helveticus H9 on spontaneously hypertensive rats. Dairy Sci Technol. 2015;95(3):321–30.

Chapter 7
Marine Shellfish Peptides and Thrombus

Ming Du, Shuzhen Cheng, Hanxiong Liu, and Huijia Yan

Abstract Thrombus is one of the major threats to human health. The prevalence of thrombosis-induced cardio-cerebrovascular diseases is increasing worldwide. According to the mechanism of thrombosis, antithrombotic drugs are divided into three categories. These categories are anticoagulants, platelet inhibitors, and fibrinolytics. Today, a large number of substances with antithrombotic activity are emerging. They aim to eliminate the unavoidable drawbacks of previously approved drugs. Such drawbacks include a high risk of bleeding and slow onset of action. Unlike drugs, food-derived functional substances are often considered to have no (or low) side effects. They are also more readily absorbed and utilized by the body. This chapter firstly describes the causes and mechanisms of thrombosis. It also provides an overview of the antithrombotic activity of bioactive peptides from marine shellfish. The screening, identification, and bioactive labeling of such bioactive peptides are also summarized. Biochemical methods, cellular models, and animal models are related to the determination of antithrombotic activity. They are also described in this chapter. In conclusion, the marine shellfish protein peptides presented in this chapter provide some new ideas. These ideas are for the prevention of thrombotic diseases. They also contribute to practical applications in the food industry.

Keywords Thrombus · Coagulation factors · Vascular endothelial cells · Marine shellfish bioactive peptides · Antithrombotic

The ocean contains abundant protein resources. It also has a balanced amino acid composition. These provide unlimited possibilities for human nutritional intake. Studies have shown that a good diet (Mediterranean diet) significantly reduces the

M. Du
College of Food Science and Engineering, Dalian Ocean University, Dalian, China

S. Cheng (✉)
School of Food Science and Technology, Dalian Polytechnic University, Dalian, China

H. Liu · H. Yan
Food Science and Engineering, Dalian Polytechnic University, Dalian, China

M. Du, S. Cheng (eds.), *Bioactive Proteins and Peptides from Marine Shellfish*,
https://doi.org/10.1007/978-981-95-3937-6_7

incidence of cardio-cerebrovascular diseases. This indicates that marine shellfish bioactive peptides have potential. They can be used in food and drug development. The goal is to prevent cardio-cerebrovascular diseases. The chapter provides an overview of the antithrombotic activity of bioactive peptides. These peptides are from marine shellfish. The screening, identification, and bioactive markers of these bioactive peptides are summarized. Biochemical methods, cellular models, and animal models are relevant to the determination of antithrombotic activity. They are described in the article. This chapter describes coagulation factors and vascular endothelial cells. It also introduces the screening and development of bioactive peptides from marine shellfish. This broadens the scope and depth of research. In vitro cellular models and in vivo animal models confirm the potential of bioactive peptides. These peptides are derived from marine shellfish. They have potential in preventing thrombosis. These peptides may inhibit the formation of fibrin clots. They do this by binding to specific coagulation factors. They may also inhibit thrombus formation by protecting vascular endothelial cells. They maintain homeostasis of the intravascular environment. Therefore, marine shellfish protein peptides are a promising source. They can be used to develop foods and drugs with antithrombotic potential.

7.1 Thrombus

Thrombus is a small solid mass. It forms in the flowing blood. Thrombus can be roughly divided into four categories. The division is based on the site, color of formation, and other conditions. These categories are white thrombus, red thrombus, mixed thrombus, and clear thrombus. The formation of thrombus is related to various factors. Such factors include vascular damage, platelet aggregation, and inflammatory reactions.

7.1.1 Thrombus and Human Health

Cardiovascular disease is the first major threat to human health. It has a high prevalence and mortality rate. It has also shown a rising trend in recent years. Cardiovascular disease remains the most common cause of death in ESC member countries. In 2021, there were more than three million deaths from it. These included over 1.6 million women and 1.5 million men. In middle-income countries, the proportion of deaths caused by cardiovascular disease is higher. It accounts for 53% of deaths in women and 46% in men. In high-income countries, this proportion is 34% and 30%, respectively [1]. Cardiovascular disease has become a major global public health issue. Most of these diseases are directly or indirectly related to thrombus formation. Examples include strokes, coronary heart disease, and lower extremity arterial disease. The prevention and treatment of thrombosis is an important way. It reduces mortality from cardiovascular disease and protects human health.

The treatment or prevention of thrombosis is not about preventing normal blood clotting in the body. It is about maintaining the dynamic balance of coagulation and dissolution in the body. The balance between blood coagulation and dissolution plays a vital role. It helps maintain the normal functioning of the body. Under normal circumstances, when a wound forms (with rupture of a blood vessel wall), blood flows outward from the wound. This happens due to blood pressure. Instead, the blood coagulates at the point where the blood vessel breaks. Its purpose is to stop blood loss from the wound. As the wound heals, the fibrinolytic system in the body dissolves the blood clot. This allows the blood vessels to return to their normal state. Blood is then normally transported throughout the body.

Since the beginning of the last century, several anticoagulant drugs have been used. They are used in the treatment of cardiovascular disease. Heparin, bivalirudin, and argatroban are all applied in various situations. These situations involve anticoagulant therapy. However, with the continuous use of drugs, side effects become increasingly apparent. For example, anticoagulation with heparin often leads to thrombocytopenia. During the process of long-term drug treatment, a discovery was made. Some patients need to keep using drugs after receiving drug anticoagulation therapy. This ensures that the disease does not recur [2]. Meanwhile, the prevalence and mortality rates of cardiovascular disease are on the rise year by year. In addition to objective factors such as population aging, other factors also contribute to the increase in its prevalence. These factors include irrational diets, unhealthy living habits, and excessive stress [3]. Therefore, it is important to focus not only on treatment, but also on how to prevent it.

7.1.2 Factors Influencing Thrombosis

The formation of thrombus is thought to be a complex process. It involves a variety of cells, proteins, and other substances. There are various ways to categorize thrombus. For example, they can be classified based on the site of formation and components of the thrombus. The categories are white thrombus, red thrombus, mixed thrombus, and clear thrombus. In 1856, German pathologist Rudolph Virchow proposed three factors. These factors are venous obstruction, vessel wall damage, and hypercoagulability. They promote thrombosis and were named the Virchow Triad [4]. As subsequent studies have advanced, the causes of thrombosis have become more numerous. But in general, they are still directly or indirectly related to these three elements. The inflammatory response can induce thrombus formation. It is often associated with endothelial damage. Generally, thrombus formation is caused by a disruption. This disruption is of the balance between clot formation and clot dissolution in the body. It often requires the involvement of coagulation factors, platelets, and vascular endothelial cells.

7.1.2.1 Coagulation Factors and Thrombosis

Plasma substances are directly involved in the blood clotting process. They are called coagulation factors. Normally, the clotting process requires the involvement of at least 14 coagulation factors. These include coagulation factors I–XIII with Roman numeral designations (excluding VI). They also include prekallikrein (PK) and high molecular weight kininogen (HMWK) in the kininogenic system. Specific information on these coagulation factors is shown in Table 7.1. Some of these factors need vitamin K for their in vivo synthesis. They are called vitamin K-dependent factors. The interaction and activation of these coagulation factors can transform fibrinogen into fibrin clots. In detail, soluble fibrinogen is converted into insoluble fibrin. This leads to the formation of fibrin clots in the blood.

However, the coagulation process is widely debated. This debate focuses on how different coagulation factors interact with each other. It also focuses on how they ultimately lead to fibrin formation. Of these debates, the classical waterfall doctrine has provided a more comprehensive explanation of the process. Briefly, the theory divides the coagulation process into three parts. These parts are the endogenous coagulation pathway, the exogenous coagulation pathway, and the common pathway. The theory also believes that the endogenous coagulation pathway is more important. The endogenous coagulation pathway involves a specific process. FXII and HMWK directly bind to negatively charged surfaces (e.g., collagen). They form FXIIa with the help of PK. FXIIa then activates FXI to form FXIa. Subsequently,

Table 7.1 Coagulation factors in humans

Factor	Synonym	Is a vitamin K-dependent factor	Relative molecular mass (KDa)	Normal plasma concentration (mg/L)
I	Fibrinogen	Not	340	2000–4000
II	Prothrombin	Yes	72	100–200
III	Tissue factor	Not	45	Extremely low (<0.1)
IV	Calcium ion	–	–	40–50
V	Mutable factor	Not	330	5–10
VII	Stabilizing factor	Yes	50	0.5–2
VIII	Antihemophilic factor	Yes	330	0.05–0.1
IX	Christmas factor	Yes	57	3–5
X	Stuart factor	Yes	56	6–10
XI	Plasma thromboplastin antecedent	Not	160	4–6
XII	Hegeman factor	Not	80	30–40
XIII	Fibrin stabilizing factor	Not	320	10–25
PK	Prekallikrein	Not	85	35–50
HMWK	High molecular weight kininogen	Not	120	70–90

FXIa activates FIX to generate FIXa. FIXa eventually activates FX to form FXa. FXa then enters the common pathway of coagulation. In contrast, the exogenous coagulation pathway begins with a specific event. It begins with the release of tissue factor (FIII). Normally, no tissue factor is present in the blood. Tissue factor is mainly derived from cells not in the blood. When a blood vessel ruptures, certain cells release tissue factor into the bloodstream. These cells include fibroblasts and smooth muscle cells. The tissue factor combines with FVIIa to form a complex. With the help of calcium ions (FIV), FX is activated to form FXa. FXa then enters the common pathway of coagulation. The exogenous coagulation pathway has a specific requirement. It only requires TF to form a complex with FVIIa. This complex forms FXa. Therefore, the formation of FXa by the exogenous coagulation pathway takes less time. This time is less than that of the endogenous coagulation pathway. After entering the common pathway, FXa performs a specific action. It cleaves prothrombin (FII) to form thrombin (FIIa). Thrombin further binds to fibrinogen to produce fibrin. Fibrin cross-links to form a spatial reticular structure. This structure marks the formation of a fibrin clot. However, clots formed by fibrin alone are unstable. Fibrin can be cleaved by FXIIIa. FXIII is activated by thrombin [5]. After this cleavage, the aggregation of fibrin monomers results in the formation of a stable clot. This stable clot is often referred to as a thrombus. The interactions between coagulation factors are shown in Fig. 7.1. Calcium ions have been omitted from the figure [6].

However, subsequent studies have found unexplained phenomena in this theory: for example, when the body lacks FXII, injecting endotoxin still causes coagulation,

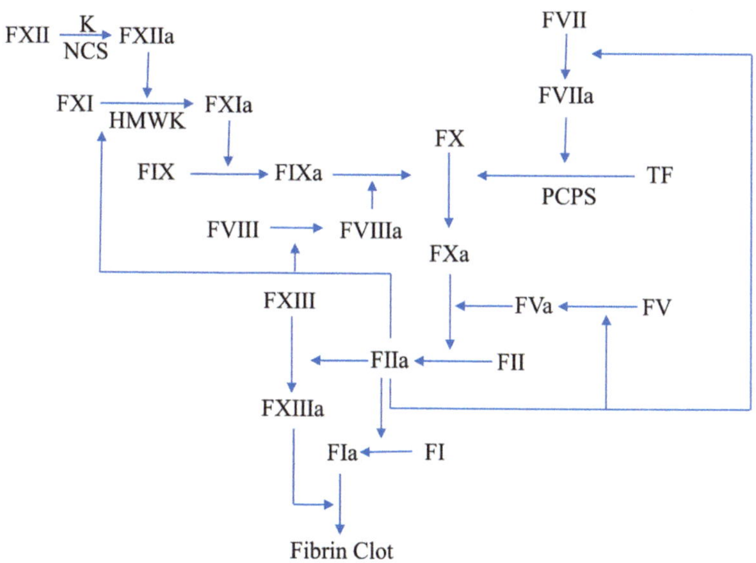

Fig. 7.1 Coagulation factor interactions in the classical waterfall doctrine. K: kallikrein; NCS: negatively charged surface; HMWK: high molecular weight kininogen; PCPS: phospholipids; TF: tissue factor

and in patients with HMWK deficiency, individuals do not have a tendency to bleed, which indicates certain problems with the classical waterfall doctrine. Therefore, building on this, a more widely recognized doctrine of coagulation process segmentation has been proposed, that is, an initiation phase followed by an amplification phase. This hypothesis suggests that blood coagulation starts with the extrinsic pathway, which then amplifies the reaction, ultimately bringing thrombin to levels sufficient to cause blood coagulation. Briefly, during the initiation phase, damaged tissue releases tissue factor into the bloodstream, which binds to FVII/FVIIa to form a complex that activates FX and generates FXa; the complex can also activate FIX to form FIXa, which binds to FVIII to form another complex that also activates FX to form FXa. Subsequently, FXa combines with FV to generate the thrombospondin complex, which cleaves thromboplastin to form thrombin (converting FII to FIIa), but due to the low activity of this complex (compared to the later-mentioned FXa-FVa complex), it only catalyzes the formation of a small amount of thrombin—insufficient to coagulate the blood. Thus, the amplification stage begins when this small amount of thrombin activates FXI to form FXIa; then, FXIa activates FIX to form FIXa, and thrombin activates FVIII to form FVIIIa. In contrast, the complex generated by FIXa and FVIIIa is highly active and can activate large amounts of FX to form FXa; finally, FXa combines with FVa (activated by thrombin) to generate the FXa-FVa complex, which catalyzes the conversion of large amounts of FII to FIIa. The quantity of this thrombin is sufficient to hydrolyze fibrinogen into fibrin and activate FXIII, which then cross-links with fibrin to form a stable clot. This process is shown in Fig. 7.2, where calcium ions, platelet surfaces, and other elements have been omitted from the figure.

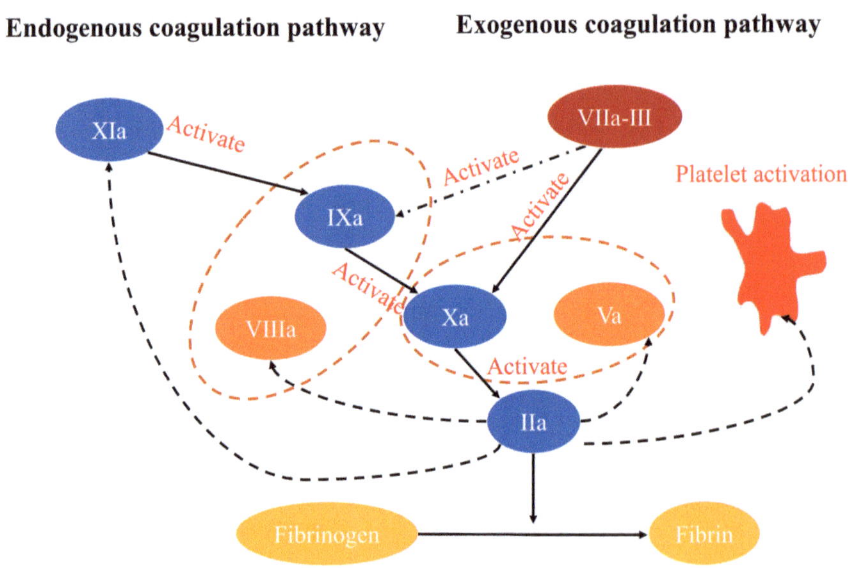

Fig. 7.2 Segmentation of the coagulation process

7.1.2.2 Platelets and Thrombus Formation

Platelets, an important component of the blood, also play a key role in blood clotting and thrombosis. During the process of thrombosis, platelets undergo deformation and aggregation; they also provide a binding surface and inhibit local fibrinolysis.

1. Platelet Activation and Aggregation
   Platelets can be activated in several ways: for example, fatty acids in the blood bind to platelet surface receptors to activate platelets; when vascular endothelial cells are damaged, the subendothelial membrane is exposed in the blood vessels, and platelets are activated by von Willebrand factor (vWF) and collagen in the blood vessels. Activated platelets undergo significant changes in morphology and function, transforming from circulating platelets (oval or disc-shaped) to dendritic platelets (extending multiple pseudopods), and their adhesion capacity is enhanced. Activated platelets can adhere to substances such as fibrinogen via integrins; at the same time, fibrinogen itself recruits activated platelets and cross-links them to adjacent activated platelets, finally enabling platelet aggregation.
2. Damaging Effects of Activated Platelets on Endothelial Cells
   When platelets are activated, they release substances such as TXA2 that can damage vascular endothelial cells; meanwhile, they also release growth factors derived from platelets to inhibit the proliferation and growth of vascular endothelial cells.
3. Platelets Inhibit Localized Fibrinolytic Reactions
   Platelets contain high concentrations of plasminogen activator inhibitor-1 (PAI-1). When platelets are activated, PAI-1 is released from within platelets to outside platelets. This leads to higher local concentrations and inhibits fibrinolytic reaction by restraining fibrinolytic enzyme formation.
4. Platelets and Coagulation Factors and Their Complexes
   Platelets can also be activated by binding to coagulation factors. Their surface receptors can combine with certain coagulation factors or provide negatively charged surfaces for coagulation factor interactions (as shown in Fig. 7.3).

7.1.2.3 Vascular Endothelial Cells and Thrombus Formation

Vascular endothelial cells are the innermost part of the blood vessel, in direct contact with the blood. They are normally arranged in a single layer with a smooth surface, which facilitates blood flow and makes it difficult for formed thrombus to adhere. Meanwhile, vascular endothelial cells act as a tissue–blood barrier; this barrier is semi-permeable and regulates the content of various substances in the blood to ensure blood homeostasis. However, when vascular endothelial cells are damaged, many changes in their properties can lead to the disruption of blood homeostasis and the formation of thrombus.

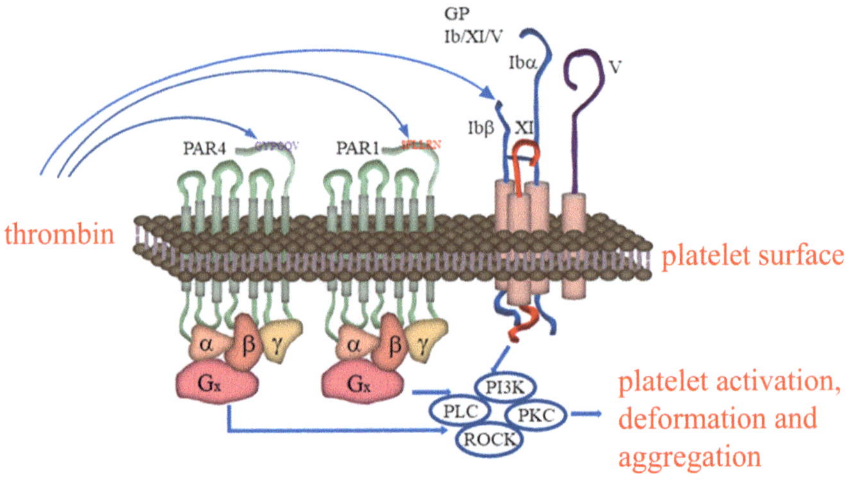

Fig. 7.3 Coagulation factors and their complexes bind to platelets resulting in platelet activation. PAR1: protease-activated receptor 1; PAR4: protease-activated receptor 4; GP Ib/IX/V: platelet membrane glycoprotein Ib/IX/V complex

1. Antithrombotic and Prothrombotic Effects of Vascular Endothelial Cells

   Under normal physiological conditions, the surface of vascular endothelial cells is smooth, making it difficult for platelets and thrombus to attach. Also, endothelial cells synthesize nitric oxide (NO) and prostacyclin (PGI2) to inhibit platelet activation. In addition, vascular endothelial cells release enzymes that promote the conversion of adenosine diphosphate (ADP) to adenosine monophosphate (AMP), thereby inhibiting platelet activation by ADP. However, when vascular endothelial cells are damaged, their function is altered. The reduction in intracellular synthesis and release of NO and PGI2, as well as a decrease in enzymes that facilitate the conversion of ADP to AMP, make platelet activation easy. At the same time, the breakdown of vascular endothelial cells results in the exposure of its underlying collagen fibers to the bloodstream, allowing platelets to be activated and providing a surface for platelet adhesion.

2. The Anticoagulant and Procoagulant Effects of Vascular Endothelial Cells

   Whether in the classical waterfall doctrine or modern coagulation theory, thrombin ultimately catalyzes fibrinogen to form fibrin, which then cross-links to form clots. In this series of processes, vascular endothelial cells play a very important role. Under normal conditions, the surface of vascular endothelial cells is smooth and flat, with no activating effect on coagulation factors and platelets. At the same time, a small amount of heparin exists in the blood; it accelerates the rate at which antithrombin-III (AT-III) inactivates thrombin. In addition, there are many receptors on the surface of vascular endothelial cells, such as thrombomodulin (TM). When thrombin binds to TM, the procoagulant activity of thrombin is lost. Meanwhile, the thrombin-TM complex can effi-

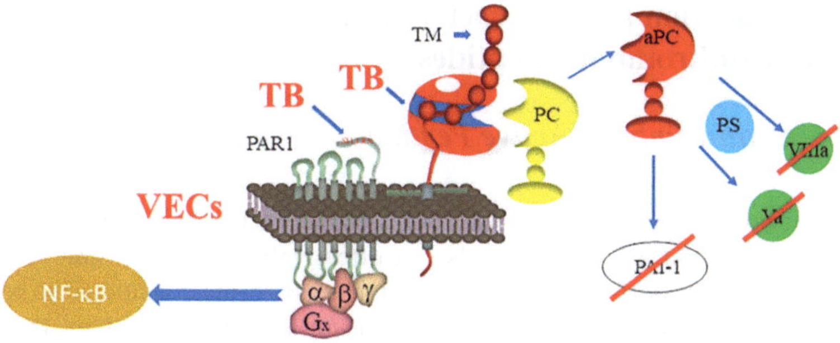

Fig. 7.4 Procoagulant and anticoagulant effects of vascular endothelial cells. VECs: vascular endothelial cells; TB: thrombin; PC: protein C; Apc: activated protein C; PS: protein S; TM: thrombomodulin; PAR1: protease-activated receptor 1; PAI-1: plasminogen activator inhibitor-1

ciently activate protein C. Activated protein C can inactivate PAI-1, thereby promoting the thrombolytic reaction. Activated protein C combined with protein S can inactivate FVa and FVIIIa, thus interrupting the coagulation reaction. When vascular endothelial cells are damaged, thrombin in the blood can bind to their surface receptor PAR1; after a series of signal transmissions, this induces an inflammatory response. Inflammatory reactions can also induce the formation of substances such as interleukins and tissue factors. Among these, tissue factor binds to FVIIa; with the help of Ca^{2+}, they can rapidly activate FX and eventually form thrombin. At the same time, vascular endothelial cells can provide a negatively charged surface for coagulation factor interactions, thereby accelerating thrombospondin activation (as shown in Fig. 7.4).

Overall, although thrombus formation is diverse, it is all related to damage to vascular endothelial cells and imbalance of blood homeostasis. Many factors can affect these processes: for example, trauma, radiation, endotoxins, nicotine, and allergic reactions can lead to vascular endothelial cell damage; vitamin K deficiency and low blood calcium levels cause abnormal interactions between coagulation factors; similarly, prolonged use of drugs such as heparin induces thrombocytopenia. All of these abnormalities can eventually imbalance blood homeostasis, leading to the formation of thrombus or other diseases. It has been over 200 years since the first effective anticoagulant heparin was used to treat deep vein thrombosis in 1916, and drugs targeting different mechanisms have been developed and utilized. However, thrombotic diseases remain "the biggest killer" threatening human health. With the deepening of research, people are increasingly aware of the limitations of drugs in treating thrombotic diseases. In recent years, more and more scholars have realized that diet and daily habits have an important impact on thrombotic diseases. Meanwhile, studies have shown that the Western diet increases cardiovascular disease morbidity and mortality compared to the Mediterranean diet, and this result is more pronounced in the elderly population [7].

7.2 Preparation and Characterization of Antithrombotic Peptides

7.2.1 Antithrombotic Active Peptide

Due to the specificity and functionality of food, active ingredients developed and obtained from food as raw materials can effectively prevent chronic diseases. Unlike drugs, food-derived functional substances are often considered to have no (or low) side effects and are more easily absorbed and utilized by the body. Therefore, many researchers have focused their attention on food, and a large number of food-derived peptides with antithrombotic activity have been reported. These peptides come from a wide range of sources, involving almost all kinds of food ingredients in our daily life. The oceans and seas occupy 70% of the earth's surface. With the world population growing and the area of land available for cultivation diminishing, the development and utilization of marine resources has become key to human development. As marine organisms live in extreme environments for long periods, they have evolved breathing and survival methods very different from those of land-based organisms to adapt to their living environment. This also leads to great variability in protein structure and amino acid sequence compared with terrestrial organisms, making aquatic products an important protein resource for screening novel antithrombotic active peptides. In daily life, we often consume shellfish, mainly including oysters, mussels, scallops, and clams. The results of available studies are summarized as follows (as shown in Table 7.2).

Table 7.2 Marine shellfish-derived antithrombotic peptides

No.	Source	Protein, peptide sequences (mixtures)	Active mechanism
1	Blue mussel	EADIDGDGQVNYEEFVAMMTSK	Coagulation factor Xa [8]
2	Blue mussel	ELEDSLDSER	Thrombin IIa [9]
3	Ark shell	HTHLQRAPHPNALGYHGK	Coagulation factor Va [10]
4	*Crassostrea gigas*	NAESLRK	Thrombin IIa [11]
5	*Crassostrea gigas*	DFEEIPEEYLQ	Thrombin IIa [12]
6	*Crassostrea gigas*	LSKEEIEEAKEV	Thrombin IIa [13]
7	*Crassostrea gigas*	IEELEEELEAER	Coagulation factor Xa, Thrombin IIa [14]
8	Green-lipped mussel	Pernin	Thrombin IIa [15]
9	Burnt-end Ark	Anticoagulant	Coagulation factor IX [16]

7.2.2 Screening Method for Antithrombotic Active Peptides

In the past, it was extremely difficult for researchers to obtain bioactive peptides from food, requiring extensive experimental operations, and the final results were sometimes unsatisfactory. The general process is as follows: identify the protein species, enzymatically or otherwise obtain a mixture of active peptides, separate and purify the active peptides step-by-step and assay for activity. Some researchers finally obtain single-component peptides, but the vast majority are still mixtures of several peptides, and finally the peptide sequences are obtained by mass spectrometry. Some researchers may synthesize the peptide sequence through chemical means and validate it, but sometimes the results are poor. Therefore, we found that traditional methods consume manpower and resources throughout the entire cycle, which is not conducive to the development and research of antithrombotic active peptides. So, we present several quick ways to screen.

7.2.2.1 Virtual Screening Based on Computer Algorithms

As bioinformatics and computer algorithms continue to evolve, researchers continue to develop new screening methods. A large number of antithrombotic bioactive peptides have been reported, and combined with the development of computer algorithms, the prediction of function and activity of unknown active peptides has been gradually realized. Predicting whether bioactive peptides bind to target proteins through molecular docking is becoming increasingly simple. The general approach is to identify the target protein to be bound and search for its 3D structure, followed by entering the information about the substance to be screened into the computer (e.g., molecular weight, amino acids). Different algorithmic procedures (e.g., flexible docking, semi-flexible docking) are used to virtually characterize and score the binding ability of the two. Finally, the strength of the activity of the substance to be verified is determined by the level of scoring or binding capacity. For example, Zheng et al. screened six substances with better inhibitory activity from the natural product database by molecular docking, using thrombin as the target protein, and all of them were verified to have better thrombin inhibitory activity in in vitro experiments [17]. The method, while fast and convenient, only predicts whether the two bind to each other or makes a preliminary determination of the strength of the ability to bind to the target protein in a series of substances; it is not possible to quantify the activity of the inhibitor.

In order to solve the above problems, constructing quantitative structure–activity relationship (QSAR) and applying it to the screening of inhibitors becomes the best way. Currently, the commonly used databases in QSAR include BIOPEP, PepBank, PeptideDB, ChEMBLE, etc. These databases include synthetic organic small molecules as well as bioactive peptides with verified efficacy, providing a good resource for QSAR modeling. Currently, the most used and more mature algorithm and validation method is 2D-QSAR. It only considers planar information such as the molecular weight of the molecule and whether it has certain special functional groups, without taking into account the spatial structure information of the molecule. This method is well suited for the quantification of small-molecule inhibitors or short-chain peptides. However, for the quantification of large molecules or inhibitors with specific spatial structures, the predictions obtained by this analytical method are usually not convincing. This is because macromolecules often have their own special spatial structures, and information such as molecular weight alone often cannot fully represent their molecular characteristics. On this basis, 3D-QSAR was developed for quantitative analysis of inhibitors. 3D-QSAR takes into account the molecular space size and the distribution of charge, which also makes the calculation results more accurate. The construction of QSAR models for thrombin, FIXa, and FXa has been reported in the literature, whereas the other coagulation factors need to be further investigated by researchers.

7.2.2.2 In Vitro Screening for Coagulation Factors

As described earlier, the formation of thrombus is related to several factors, and among them coagulation factors play a crucial role. At the same time, since coagulation factors mostly function in the blood and the techniques for obtaining different coagulation factors are becoming increasingly sophisticated, most researchers use coagulation factors as antithrombotic targets. At present, commonly used coagulation factors for targets include FIIa and FXa/FX, and there are also some studies on other coagulation factors such as FXIa and FIXa. For different research purposes, various methods will be introduced for rapid in vitro screening and target protein localization.

1. Activated Partial Thromboplastin Time (APTT)/Prothrombin Time (PT) Method

   This method is two of the four routine tests of the coagulation system. Originally used to detect the presence of coagulation abnormalities in the blood, it has been improved to become a rapid screening method for anticoagulant activity in vitro. The method follows the classical waterfall doctrine, which divides coagulation factors into endogenous coagulation pathways, exogenous coagulation pathways, and common pathways, and both need to be tested at the same time to have some significance. Among these, only APTT prolongation represents an inhibitor interacting with one or more factors in the endogenous coagulation pathway; PT prolongation represents an inhibitor interacting with one or more factors in the exogenous coagulation pathway; when both are prolonged, it represents an inhibitor interacting with one or more factors in the common pathway. The advantage of this method is that it can quickly narrow down the target protein for inhibitors with unknown activity; meanwhile, the method is simple and convenient, and is suitable for samples with color in the solution, so it has wide applicability. However, the disadvantage of this method is that, although it can narrow down the range of target proteins, it is not yet possible to accurately localize the specific target proteins.

2. Chromogenic Substrate Method

   This method takes advantage of the fact that some coagulation factors have enzyme-catalyzed properties, which can specifically recognize the substrate and catalyze its hydrolysis. The chromogenic substrate is a synthetic small molecule. Under normal conditions, the aqueous solution is colorless and transparent. When hydrolyzed by the corresponding coagulation factor, the free p-nitroaniline (pNA) appears yellow in solution. Moreover, the absorbance values were positively correlated with the enzyme activity under the same conditions. Therefore, it is possible to rapidly detect whether an inhibitor has an inhibitory effect on a specific coagulation factor by using an enzyme marker. Also, more conclusions can be drawn if a standard curve is plotted. The method is fast, accurate and simple. However, the limitations of the chromogenic substrate result in the method not being applicable to all coagulation factors. For coagulation factors that act as cofactors and do not have catalytic properties, the method cannot be applied. Currently the method is mainly used for FIIa, FXa, FXIa & FXIIa, and the corresponding color-emitting substrates are S-2238, S-2222/S-2765, S-2366 & S-2302, respectively.

7.3 Activity and Mechanism of Antithrombotic Peptides

Thrombus formation is associated with coagulation factor abnormalities, platelet activation, and endothelial cell injury. Most researchers have targeted the search for a bioactive peptide that can inhibit coagulation factor activity; a few researchers have also focused their antithrombotic efforts on inhibiting platelet activation and aggregation or promoting endothelial cell repair and proliferation. In order to facilitate the exploration of the activity characterization and specific antithrombotic mechanisms of bioactive peptides, this chapter will be presented from three different perspectives.

7.3.1 Physical and Chemical Methods

Physicochemical methods are mainly used to characterize and mechanistically analyze the antithrombotic properties of bioactive peptides under in vitro conditions. Since most studies have focused their targets on coagulation factors, the methods used are mostly characterization of protein–peptide interactions. Common methods are shown in Table 7.3.

Table 7.3 Common physical and chemical research methods

Methods	Focal point	Advantages	Disadvantages
Fibrinogen time method	Effect of inhibitors on thrombin-induced fibrinogen coagulation	Fast and simple, it is suitable for the characterization of not only thrombin catalytic site inhibitors but also thrombin exosite-I inhibitors.	This method is only suitable for the characterization of thrombin inhibitors and is prone to produce false-positive results for other coagulation factors or substances that interfere with normal fibrin aggregation.
Fluorescence method	Structural changes in the binding of the two or the dynamics of the labeled molecules in the complexes	It is sensitive and has low reagent consumption. It can easily reveal the local structure of the medium and the dynamic properties of the labeled molecules.	Not applicable to some autofluorescent substances, mostly requires dye labeling, but the dye may interfere with the binding of the two.
Circular dichroism (CD) spectroscopy	Effects of interactions on protein (or peptide) secondary structure	The effect of interactions on the secondary structure of protein (or peptide). Fast, accurate, extremely sensitive, and does not require other substances to be labeled to reflect the interaction between the two in solution.	High purity is required and some impurities (e.g., aromatic polysaccharides) can affect the experimental results.
Surface plasmon resonance and biosphere interference techniques	Molecular-level interactions	High sensitivity, small sample size, mathematical modeling to derive the two binding constants, etc.	Requires immobilization of one of the molecules, which may affect the binding of both, and is insensitive to weak binding.
Isothermal titration calorimetry	Thermodynamic parameters related to molecular interactions	Direct collection of thermodynamic parameters, including binding constants, stoichiometry of binding sites, free energy (ΔG), entropy (ΔH), and enthalpy change (ΔS); unlabeled and does not affect interactions.	Sample purity requirements are high, and samples with weak binding capacity or slow exotherm are difficult to characterize. The experiment time is long, and there is a certain requirement for sample stability.

(continued)

Table 7.3 (continued)

Methods	Focal point	Advantages	Disadvantages
Microscopic imaging methods (cryo-electron microscopy, atomic force microscopy, transmission electron microscopy, etc.)	Molecular micro/ macro morphological changes	Directly observe the effect of inhibitors on thrombus formation (coagulation) and even obtain 3D structures of molecular interactions. The 3D structures are obtained by freezing under solution conditions, so the interaction information obtained is closer to the real situation.	Some methods may require labeling or staining, which may affect the results of molecular interactions. For smaller molecules, it is difficult to obtain 3D structures.
X-ray crystal diffraction	Molecular interactions, aggregation, and structural information	Without labeling, the interaction mechanism of the molecules after the formation of crystals was analyzed to confirm the binding site and 3D structure.	It is not suitable for molecules that are difficult to culture to obtain crystals, nor for molecules that a larger ratio flexible. For some proteins, the addition of a suitable ligand is required to stabilize the structure. Since the molecules are in the crystalline state rather than the solution state during analysis, the most realistic binding mechanism for reactive molecules may not be possible.
Computer simulation	Information on molecular interactions under virtual conditions	Fast and convenient, without the need for actual experimental operation. Molecules can be completed in a short period of time, which can provide reference information for the direction of subsequent experiments and provide a preliminary basis for the study of molecular action mechanisms.	The simulation results differ from the actual results and need to be verified and confirmed by subsequent experiments. For an unknown molecule, more time is usually required.

7.3.1.1 The Fibrinogen Clotting Time Method

The fibrinogen clotting time (FCT) method is a simple and rapid method for determining whether an inhibitor has thrombin inhibitory activity. Thrombin specifically recognizes fibrinogen and cleaves it to form fibrin, resulting in solution coagulation. FCT results are negatively correlated with thrombin activity, that is, the stronger the thrombin activity, the shorter the FCT. The FCT method has a wider range of applications than the chromogenic substrate method; it can detect whether the inhibitor binds to the thrombin catalytic site and external site-1. The main disadvantage of this method is that calcium ion chelators also have a significant effect on prolonging the coagulation time (calcium ions are required for the coagulation of fibrin). Therefore, this method requires attention to the calcium ion concentration in the entire solution system to avoid false-positive results.

7.3.1.2 Spectral Analysis

Spectroscopic methods are commonly used to study the interaction between inhibitors and target proteins. The simplest and most commonly used methods are CD and fluorescence spectroscopy. The interaction between an inhibitor and a target protein will change its structure; therefore, by comparing the structural changes of the target protein before and after the addition of the inhibitor, it can be determined whether they bind. Structural changes can also lead to energy changes, which can cause fluorescence bursts; thus, measuring the fluorescence energy intensity before and after the reaction can also determine whether they are bound together. This type of assay is extremely sensitive but has many shortcomings: it is not possible to explore the mechanism of action, and it cannot be used for the study of autofluorescent substances.

In addition to these two methods, surface plasma resonance (SPR) and bio-layer interferometry (BLI) have been used to study the interaction between thrombin and inhibitors. As an emerging technology, BLI determines whether two substances can interact with each other through the phenomenon of light interference. When molecule A is stably immobilized on the sensor, it increases the thickness of the sensor; the change in thickness creates a difference in the optical path of the interfering light, and this signal difference is recorded. The sensor with immobilized molecule A is inserted into a solution of molecule B at the appropriate concentration; when the two are combined, the thickness and density change, and the optical path difference changes again, which is also recorded. When there is no interaction between the two, the optical path difference does not change, so no new signals are recorded. The entire experiment is usually performed in less than an hour, making it possible to quickly and accurately characterize whether the two are interacting. In addition, when a gradient concentration is set for the molecule, the affinity constants of the two substances can also be analyzed with the appropriate program. Similarly, SPR can be used to characterize and infer affinity constants. Although both methods can be extremely accurate and calculate affinity constants, the high cost of experimental consumables negatively impacts their large-scale application. In addition, for weakly bound inhibitors, the affinity constants derived by these methods are often not accurate enough and need to be co-characterized or validated by other methods.

7.3.1.3 Isothermal Titrimetric Calorimetry

Isothermal titrimetric calorimetry is a widely used classical method of thermodynamics for determining whether two substances are bound together. By analyzing the curve fit of the titration results, information such as the binding constant (K), stoichiometry (n), and enthalpy change (ΔH) of the reaction system can be obtained. Further analysis of these parameters can infer the main types of bonds formed when the two bind to each other. This information can be used as a basis for speculating the binding mode of the inhibitor to the target protein, which is a good guide for other experiments. In the experiment, other heat-absorbing or exothermic reactions and even vibrations in the environment can affect the results; thus, the method has higher requirements for the purity and concentration of the substance to be measured. In addition, due to the long stirring time of the whole experiment, it also has higher requirements on the stability of the test object. Combined with amino acid site-directed mutagenesis techniques, we can find out the key amino acids that affect the binding ability of the inhibitor. The fact that the method does not require secondary labeling or chemical modification and can realistically characterize the binding state of the reactants has led to its widespread use.

7.3.1.4 Microscopic Imaging Methods

Microscopic imaging methods have two main roles in the study of the interaction of coagulation factors and their inhibitors: one is to characterize the inhibitory effect of inhibitors on coagulation factors, and the other is to analyze the action mechanism of inhibitors. The former mainly characterizes the process by which a particular coagulation factor interacts with an inhibitor (or other substance) and studies the strength of the inhibitor activity. Some investigators have been able to visualize the effect of inhibitors on thrombin-induced fibrinogen aggregation by comparing the difference in thrombin-induced fibrinogen aggregation with and without inhibitors. Most of the metrics can be characterized when using this type of method, such as the diameter of fiber bundles formed by fibrin cross-linking and the degree of platelet activation. In contrast, another method is more straightforward. Cryo-electron microscopy, a new technique, is now widely used for structural analysis, so this technique can also be used to directly analyze the structure of inhibitor-target protein complexes and study their mechanisms of action. However, in the current state of the technique, this method can only be used to resolve some large molecular weight substances, such as protein–protein complexes. Since this method freezes and images complex solutions, it provides a true image of the bound state of the reacting substances in solution.

In addition to cryo-electron microscopy techniques, X-ray crystal diffraction techniques can also be used to obtain the crystal structure of the composite. When using this method, the inhibitor and thrombin complexes need to be crystallized and then diffracted to collect spectra to obtain the structure. As a result, it is usually easier to obtain structural information and analyze the mechanism of action for compounds that can be easily crystallized; however, it is somewhat difficult to use this method for some compounds that are difficult to crystallize or are unstable. In addition, since this method analyzes the complex after crystallization and the cryo-electron microscopic treatment of the complex is completely different, the crystal structures obtained by the two methods are different. These two methods have their own advantages and disadvantages: cryo-electron microscopy can better reflect the real state of the interaction between the two, but the ability to analyze small molecule complexes is slightly insufficient; while X-ray diffraction technique can obtain the crystal structure of small molecules, but it is difficult to obtain the structure of complexes that are more flexible or difficult to crystallize.

7.3.1.5 Computer Simulation

In addition, computer simulation methods such as molecular docking and molecular dynamics are increasingly being used to explore the binding mechanism of inhibitors to thrombin. Nowadays, computer simulation can be used to explore the mechanism of action; in addition to molecular docking and molecular dynamics, means such as amino acid virtual mutation are also used. Therefore, a comprehensive and in-depth study of its mechanism can be carried out. Although the results of simulation still need to be confirmed by actual experiments, the rational use of this method can save a lot of resources and provide guidance for subsequent experiments.

7.3.2 Cell Model

Since platelets do not possess a nuclear structure, most of the research surrounding thrombosis has focused on vascular endothelial cells. Since the cells themselves do not have the ability to form thrombus, they also work together with coagulation factors and platelets to form thrombus in the body. And the experimental methods are mostly peptide and exogenous stimulants acting together on endothelial cells to detect the effect on the normal function of endothelial cells, so they are not described too much in this section.

7.3.3 Animal Model

Studies on food-borne bioactive peptides often show significant in vitro results and unsatisfactory in vivo results. This is closely related to their source and the strength of their targeting ability. In many cases, bioactive peptides are digested into shorter peptides or amino acids in the digestive tract, thus losing their functional activity. Therefore, the results of animal experiments are particularly important in the study. Here, we introduce several common and simple animal experimental methods to verify the antithrombotic ability of bioactive peptides.

7.3.3.1 Mice Tail Thrombosis

The method can be applied to rats or mice. The principle is that the blood vessel endothelium is damaged by chemical agents such as carrageenan or other means, and then thrombi are formed [18]. The thinness of the blood vessels in the tail of the rat and the slower flow of blood allow the thrombi formed to accumulate in the tail. Thrombus formation was observed in the rat tail within 24–72 h after the experiment. By comparing the length of the thrombus in different groups, the antithrombotic ability of the inhibitor can be determined. The advantages of this method are that the phenomenon is obvious, the operation is simple, and the animals are not lethal. The disadvantages of this method are that the differences between individuals are large, and the requirements for the experimental environment are high. The experimental period is long.

7.3.3.2 Acute Pulmonary Embolism

Liu et al. successfully induced acute pulmonary embolism in mice using thrombin [19]. The antithrombotic peptide activity was determined by observing the mortality and disability rates of the mice. The advantage of this method is that the experimental effect is obvious and the experimental period is very short (usually 5–10 min). The disadvantages of this method are that the experimental individuals will die and the cost of the experiment is high; moreover, because the experimental phenomenon appears quickly, it is often necessary to be injected, which is quite different from practical application.

7.3.3.3 Tail Cutting

The tail-cutting method was used to determine the antithrombotic and anticoagulant ability of the bioactive peptides. The tails of experimental rats were cut at 0.3–0.5 cm from the end of the tails, and then the tails were placed in a water bath at 37 °C to observe the time required for natural coagulation. The antithrombotic and anticoagulant ability of the bioactive peptide was determined by comparing the time duration of different groups. The advantage of this method is that there are various ways of peptide administration, and the individuals do not die after the experiment. The disadvantages of this method are that there are large individual differences, and the way of tail cutting, angle, and environmental factors may interfere with the results of the experiment.

7.3.3.4 Clot Weighing

This method is often used in larger animals such as rats and rabbits. The principle is to damage the blood vessels by different methods (e.g., ferric chloride embolization, hydrogen peroxide embolization) [20], remove the clots after a certain period of time and wash it, and finally weigh the embolus. By comparing the weights of different groups of clots, the strength of the peptide antithrombotic ability was determined. The method is reproducible and can be combined with other materials to induce targeted thrombosis (e.g., arterial thrombosis, venous thrombosis). There are various ways to administer the drug. The disadvantage is that it requires a high level of skill on the part of the experimenter, and most individuals die after the experiment. The cost of the experiment is high.

Overall, these several animal experimental methods introduced are unable to study the mechanism of action of antithrombotic peptides in depth. However, this has an irreplaceable role in the subsequent development and application of peptides. At the same time, only through animal experiments can we further find out the dosage of the peptide in the future practical application.

7.4 Summary

Cardiovascular and cerebrovascular diseases, as the top threat to human health, still require significant efforts in their treatment. However, as a chronic metabolic disease, more and more studies show that daily diet and lifestyle have a significant impact on the prevalence. Therefore, how to achieve early and effective prevention has become a problem that needs to be solved nowadays. In this chapter, the mechanisms of blood coagulation and thrombosis in normal human body are briefly introduced, and the current research directions for this type of disease are also pointed out. In order to better characterize the targets and activities of the active substances, a variety of experimental methods in vivo and in vitro are introduced to provide reference for researchers.

References

1. Timmis A, Aboyans V, Vardas P, Townsend N, Torbica A, Kavousi M, Boriani G, Huculeci R, Kazakiewicz D, Scherr D, Karagiannidis E, Cvijic M, Kapłon-Cieślicka A, Ignatiuk B, Raatikainen P, De Smedt D, Wood A, Dudek D, Van Belle E, Weidinger F, Societies, E. S. C. N. C. European Society of Cardiology: the 2023 atlas of cardiovascular disease statistics. Eur Heart J. 2024;45(38):4019–62.
2. Kyrle PA, Rosendaal FR, Eichinger S. Risk assessment for recurrent venous thrombosis. Lancet. 2010;376(9757):2032–9.
3. Chandra P, Bhave R. Assessing the risk factors associated with cardiovascular disease. Eur J Prev Cardiol. 2018;25(9):932–3.
4. Galanaud JP, Laroche JP, Righini M. The history and historical treatments of deep vein thrombosis. J Thromb Haemost. 2013;11(3):402–11.
5. Alshehri FSM, Whyte CS, Mutch NJ. Factor XIII-A: an indispensable "factor" in haemostasis and wound healing. Int J Mol Sci. 2021;22(6):3055.
6. Cheng S, Tu M, Liu H, Zhao G, Du M. Food-derived antithrombotic peptides: preparation, identification, and interactions with thrombin. Crit Rev Food Sci Nutr. 2019;59(sup1):S81–95.
7. Evoy CM, Neville C, Temple NJ, Woodside JV. Effect of diet on vascular health. Rev Clin Gerontol. 2014;24(1):25–40.
8. Jung WK, Kim SK. Isolation and characterisation of an anticoagulant oligopeptide from blue mussel, Mytilus edulis. Food Chem. 2009;117(4):687–92.
9. Qiao M, Tu M, Wang Z, Mao F, Chen H, Qin L, Du M. Identification and antithrombotic activity of peptides from blue mussel (*Mytilus edulis*) protein. Int J Mol Sci. 2018;19(1):138.
10. Jung WK, Jo HY, Qian ZJ, Jeong YJ, Park SG, Choi IW, Kim SK. A novel anticoagulant protein with high affinity to blood coagulation factor Va from Tegillarca granosa. J Biochem Mol Biol. 2007;40(5):832–8.
11. Cheng S, Tu M, Liu H, An Y, Du M, Zhu B. A novel heptapeptide derived from Crassostrea gigas shows anticoagulant activity by targeting for thrombin active domain. Food Chem. 2021;334:127507.
12. Cheng S, Tu M, Chen H, Xu Z, Wang Z, Liu H, Zhao G, Zhu B, Du M. Identification and inhibitory activity against α-thrombin of a novel anticoagulant peptide derived from oyster (*Crassostrea gigas*) protein. Food Funct. 2018;9(12):6391–400.
13. Chen H, Cheng S, Fan F, Tu M, Xu Z, Du M. Identification and molecular mechanism of antithrombotic peptides from oyster proteins released in simulated gastro-intestinal digestion. Food Funct. 2019;10(9):5426–35.
14. Cheng S, Wu D, Liu H, Xu X, Zhu B, Du M. A novel anticoagulant peptide discovered from Crassostrea gigas by combining bioinformatics with the enzymolysis strategy: inhibitory kinetics and mechanisms. Food Funct. 2021;12(20):10136–46.
15. Scotti PD, Dearing SC, Greenwood DR, Newcomb RD. Pernin: a novel, self-aggregating haemolymph protein from the New Zealand green-lipped mussel, Perna canaliculus (Bivalvia: *Mytilidae*). Comp Biochem Physiol B Biochem Mol Biol. 2001;128(4):767–79.
16. Jung W-K, Je J-Y, Kim H-J, Kim S-K. A novel anticoagulant protein from Scapharca broughtonii. BMB Rep. 2002;35(2):199–205.
17. Zheng X, Pu P, Ding B, Bo W, Qin D, Liang G. Identification of the functional food ingredients with antithrombotic properties via virtual screen and experimental studies. Food Chem. 2021;362:130237.
18. Ma N, Yang Y, Liu X, Li S, Qin Z, Li J. Plasma metabonomics and proteomics studies on the anti-thrombosis mechanism of aspirin eugenol ester in rat tail thrombosis model. J Proteome. 2020;215:103631.
19. Liu H, Tu M, Cheng S, Xu Z, Xu X, Du M. Anticoagulant decapeptide interacts with thrombin at the active site and exosite-I. J Agric Food Chem. 2020;68(1):176–84.
20. Shaya SA, Gani DM, Weitz JI, Kim PY, Gross PL. Factor XIII prevents pulmonary emboli in mice by stabilizing deep vein thrombi. Thromb Haemost. 2019;119(6):992–9.

Chapter 8
Marine Shellfish Peptides and Gout

Ming Du, Zhen Yuan, Peiting Lv, Shuzhen Cheng, and Xiaoyu Ma

Abstract Gout, a metabolic disease, has increased steadily in prevalence worldwide, particularly among men and in regions with high socio-demographic index (SDI) values. The development of gout is strongly associated with hyperuricemia, a precursor condition. Currently, treatment options for gout and hyperuricemia are limited. The primary medications for both conditions fall into two categories: those that promote uric acid excretion and those that block uric acid formation. Both medication classes are frequently associated with a range of adverse effects. Therefore, it is particularly important to find new treatment methods. Xanthine oxidase (XO) is one of the key enzymes regulating uric acid production, and xanthine oxidase inhibitory peptides derived from marine shellfish show potential applications in this field. Small-molecule peptides may be more likely to have an inhibitory impact on XO. Peptides with xanthine oxidase inhibitors (XOI) action have been effectively isolated from a range of marine creatures. These peptides are predominantly neutral or slightly basic and commonly contain specific amino acid residues such as tryptophan (Trp). This chapter describes the preparation, isolation, purification, identification, and characterization of XO inhibitory peptides, and discusses their potential applications in treating gout and hyperuricemia. Though research into XO inhibitory peptides derived specifically from marine shellfish is still limited, existing studies offer both a theoretical basis and practical guidance for developing bioactive peptides from marine shellfish proteins.

Keywords Marine shellfish peptide · Gout · Hyperuricemia · Xanthine oxidase inhibitory peptide

---

M. Du
College of Food Science and Engineering, Dalian Ocean University, Dalian, China

Z. Yuan
Resource and Environment, Shanxi Agricultural University, Jinzhong, China

P. Lv · X. Ma
Food Science and Engineering, Dalian Polytechnic University, Dalian, China

S. Cheng (✉)
School of Food Science and Technology, Dalian Polytechnic University, Dalian, China

M. Du, S. Cheng (eds.), *Bioactive Proteins and Peptides from Marine Shellfish*,
https://doi.org/10.1007/978-981-95-3937-6_8

Gout is a painful and episodic inflammatory disease caused by excessive purine metabolism or impaired uric acid excretion. Hyperuricemia represents the initial stage of gout. XO is the key enzyme regulating uric acid production during purine metabolism. Inhibiting XO activity reduces uric acid production, thereby alleviating hyperuricemia. Existing therapeutic drugs are associated with various side effects. In contrast, protein-derived small-molecule uric acid-lowering peptides have attracted significant research interest due to their low preparation cost, high safety, ease of absorption, potent activity, stability, and specificity. This chapter introduces the incidence, progression, and pathogenesis of gout and hyperuricemia, and summarizes the mechanisms of action and side effects of therapeutic drugs used at different disease stages. Methods for the isolation, purification, screening, and activity analysis of XO inhibitory peptides are described.

8.1 Gout and Purine Metabolism

8.1.1 Prevalence of Gout and Hyperuricemia

With rising living standards, dietary changes, and increased life expectancy, gout has become the second most prevalent metabolic disease in China after diabetes mellitus [1]. Global gout epidemiology data from 2020 reveal a gradual worldwide increase in gout incidence in recent years. The prevalence of hyperuricemia ranges from 2.6% to 36.0%, and the prevalence of gout ranges from 0.03% to 15.30% among people of different races. Both conditions show significant increases and are affecting younger populations [2]. Gout prevalence is higher in men than women and increases linearly with age until 64 years. Additionally, prevalence correlates with SDI values. Gout risk is three times higher in high-SDI areas than in low-SDI areas. Projections indicate gout-related mortality may increase by 55% by 2060 [3]. Gout attacks involve severe joint pain [4]. Although the pain is self-limiting [5], severe cases can lead to joint deformity and dysfunction. Complications pose a significant concern in gout. Among gout patients, it is quite common to encounter conditions such as cardiovascular disease, diabetes mellitus, obesity, and chronic kidney disease [6].

8.1.2 Course and Pathogenesis of Gout and Hyperuricemia

8.1.2.1 Course of Gout and Hyperuricemia

Gout is a painful condition characterized by recurrent inflammatory episodes. This recurrent inflammatory disease results from excessive purine metabolism or impaired uric acid excretion [4]. The disease progression is illustrated in Fig. 8.1. Gout and hyperuricemia represent distinct phases of the same pathological

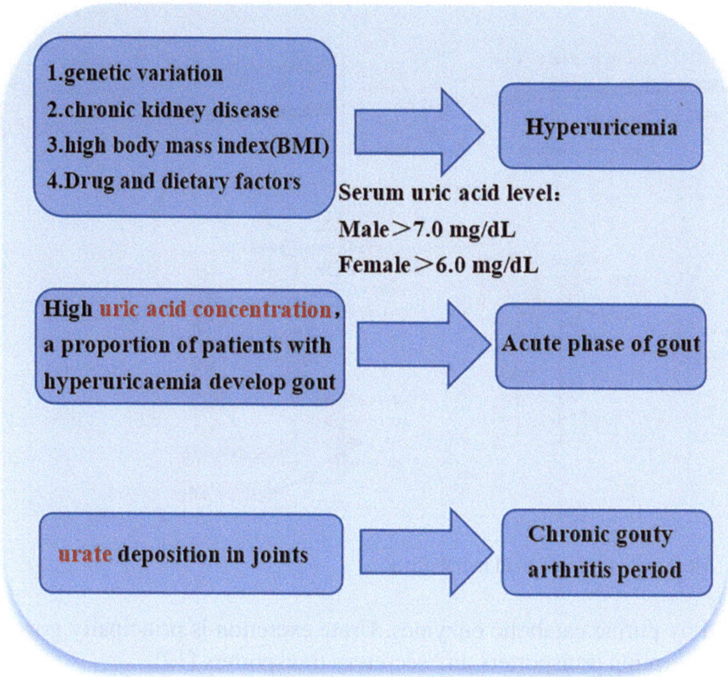

Fig. 8.1 Course of gout onset

spectrum [7]. Gout prevalence remains significantly lower than hyperuricemia prevalence, though the underlying reasons are incompletely understood [6]. Hyperuricemia constitutes the initial stage preceding gout attacks and arises from multiple factors, including genetic variants, chronic kidney disease, high body mass index, medications, and dietary factors [8]. While hyperuricemia is a prerequisite for gout, only a subset of hyperuricemia individuals develop clinical gout [6]. Clinical hyperuricemia diagnosis requires serum uric acid levels exceeding 7.0 mg/dL in men or 6.0 mg/dL in women [9]. Persistently elevated uric acid concentrations trigger acute gout phases characterized by intermittent attacks and progressively prolonged symptomatic periods [7]. Monosodium urate (MSU) crystals deposit systemically, predominantly periarticularly, forming tophi [10] that progress to chronic gouty arthritis [7, 10].

8.1.2.2 The Pathogenesis of Gout

Serum uric acid levels directly correlate with gout development. Elevated serum uric acid levels result from either increased urate production or decreased renal excretion. Both the magnitude and duration of hyperuricemia determine gout progression risk [11]. As shown in Fig. 8.2, endogenous urate production is primarily

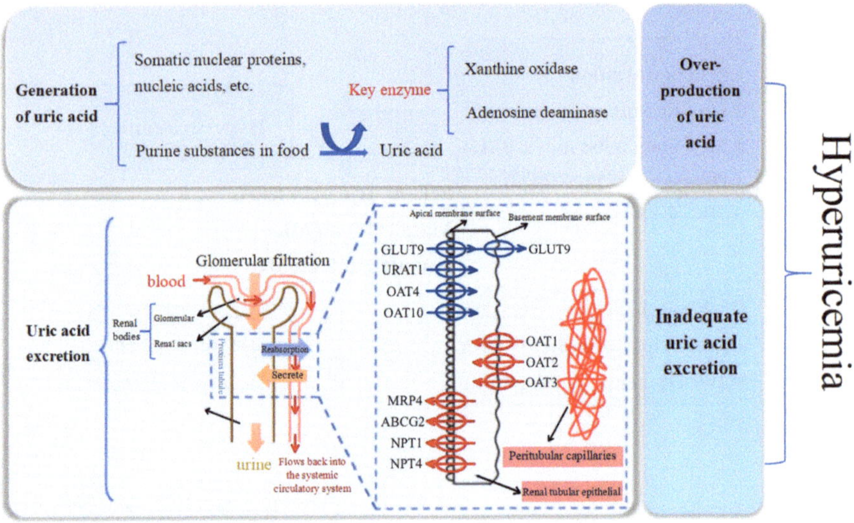

Fig. 8.2 Mechanisms of uric acid metabolism

regulated by purine catabolic enzymes. Urate excretion is principally governed by urate reabsorption transporters and secretory transporters [12].

Adenosine deaminase (ADA) and XO constitute the key regulatory enzymes in the purine-to-uric acid metabolic pathway. ADA, a sulfhydryl-containing enzyme, catalyzes the deamination of adenosine to inosine. Purine nucleoside phosphorylase (PNP) subsequently cleaves inosine to generate hypoxanthine. XO ultimately oxidizes hypoxanthine to xanthine, then xanthine to uric acid [13].

As shown in Fig. 8.2, uric acid is excreted primarily by the kidneys. It enters the renal tubules after glomerular filtration. It is reabsorbed and resecreted in the proximal tubules of the renal tubules [14]. If the body expresses abnormal uric acid reabsorption proteins or secretory proteins, resulting in increased reabsorption or decreased excretion of uric acid, hyperuricemia will result. At present, a variety of reabsorption proteins and secreted proteins have been found in the apical membrane surface and the basal membrane surface of the proximal renal tubules. Uric acid reabsorption proteins include URAT1, GLUT9, OAT4, and OAT10. Uric acid secretory proteins include OAT1, OAT2, OAT3, MRP4, NPT1, NPT4, and ABCG2 [8, 12, 15–17].

8.1.3 Treatment of Gout and Hyperuricemia

At present, gout cannot be cured. Management primarily focuses on controlling serum urate levels and preventing acute arthritis attacks. This approach prevents urate deposition, tophi formation, and renal impairment. Drugs to reduce blood uric acid mainly include drugs that promote uric acid excretion and inhibit uric acid production [18], as shown in Table 8.1. Acute inflammatory gout attacks require

Table 8.1 Drugs used to treat gout

	Name of the drug	Mechanism	Side effects	References
Drugs that promote uric acid efflux	Probenecid	Inhibition of URAT1 and GLUT9.	Chills, fever, rash, myalgia, shortness of breath, nausea, vomiting, and vasomotor failure that develop from allergies.	[19–21]
	Benzbromarone	Inhibition of URAT1 and GLUT9.	Abnormal liver function, severe hepatitis, and liver failure.	[19, 22]
	Sulfinpyrazone	Inhibition of URAT1.	Negative effects on renal function and its adverse pharmacological effects.	[23]
	Lesinurad	Inhibition of URAT1 and OAT4.	1. Headache, gastroesophageal reflux disease, and infection. 2. Lesinurad at a single therapeutic dose ≥400 mg can increase serum creatinine levels 1.5–2 times or cause acute renal failure.	[24, 25]
Drugs that inhibit the production of uric acid	Allopurinol	Xanthine oxidase inhibitors.	Nausea, vomiting, taste changes, drowsiness, diarrhea, and elevated transaminases. The complication is allopurinol anaphylaxis syndrome (AHS), characterized by Stevens–Johnson syndrome and toxic epidermal necrolysis, eosinophilia, leukocytosis, fever, hepatitis, and renal failure.	[26–29]
	Febuxostat	Xanthine oxidase inhibitors.	Muscle aches, stomachache, headache, rash, diarrhea, and mildly elevated liver enzymes were noted.	[22, 28, 29]
	Topiroxostat	Xanthine oxidase inhibitors.	Polyarthritis, nasopharyngitis, and elevated liver enzymes.	[22]

(continued)

Table 8.1 (continued)

	Name of the drug	Mechanism	Side effects	References
Drugs that treat the inflammation of gout	Colchicine	Inhibits caspase-1 activation, thereby preventing IL-1β production and inflammatory vesicle activation. Also prevents neutrophil traveling and activity, which can cause gout symptoms.	The side effects are substantial and dose-dependent. Excessive doses can lead to toxic effects, including gastrointestinal reactions, liver and kidney damage, and even death in adults.	[28–30]
	Nonsteroidal anti-inflammatory drugs (NSAIDs)	Blocking the conversion of arachidonic acid into prostate by inhibiting the cyclooxygenase COX, thereby achieving anti-inflammatory and analgesic effects.	At therapeutic doses, NSAIDs can cause liver and kidney damage, neurological, urinary and hematological abnormalities, gastrointestinal lesions and bleeding, increased blood pressure, myocardial infarction, or failure.	[31]
	Corticosteroids	Reduces the activation, proliferation, and survival of a variety of inflammatory cells. Reduces the migration of neutrophils and inhibits prostaglandins and proinflammatory cytokines such as IL-1β.	When patients stop using hormone drugs, rebound phenomenon is easy to occur, and long-term use is easy to lead to adrenocortical hyperfunction, cardiovascular disease, and osteoporosis.	[13, 32]
Recombinant uricase	Pegloticase	Breaks down uric acid into the more water-soluble allantoin, which is easily removed through the kidneys.	Common adverse reactions included rash, dyspnea, and hot flashes, most of which could be relieved spontaneously.	[33, 34]
	Rasburicase	Breaks down uric acid into the more water-soluble allantoin, which is easily removed through the kidneys.	Complex allergic reactions, including bronchospasm or skin reactions, especially after repeated infusions.	[35]

rapid anti-inflammatory treatment for pain and inflammation control. It can also be treated with the enzyme uricase, which is not found in the human body. Drugs that promote uric acid excretion include probenecid, benzbromarone, sulfinpyrazone, and lesinurad. Drugs that inhibit uric acid production include allopurinol, febuxostat, and topiroxostat. Drugs for the treatment of inflammation in gout include colchicine, nonsteroidal anti-inflammatory drugs (NSAIDs), and corticosteroids. Recombinant uricase drugs include Pegloticase and Rasburicase. Current gout medications frequently cause significant adverse effects (Table 8.1). Studies demonstrate that flavonoids, phenolic acids, terpenoids, and alkaloids exhibit urate-lowering potential. However, prohibitive extraction costs limit industrial applications of these natural compounds. Protein-derived small-molecule uric acid-lowering peptides have attracted the attention of researchers due to their low preparation cost, safety, easy absorption, high activity, stability, and specificity. Certain peptides demonstrate both in vitro xanthine oxidase inhibition and in vivo urate reduction. Therefore, the development of food-sourced, novel, low-toxicity uric acid-lowering active substances is of great importance.

8.2 Preparation and Identification of Xanthine Oxidase Inhibitory Peptides

Current urate-lowering research primarily focuses on screening XOI [36]. These inhibitors bind to the catalytically active site in the center of molybdenum cofactor (molybdopterin, Mo-pt). Reversibly or irreversibly inhibits xanthine oxidase activity and prevents hydroxylation of substrates. This reduces uric acid production and lowers the concentration of uric acid in the serum to achieve the effect of treating high uric acid.

Notably, xanthine oxidase inhibitory peptides from marine shellfish remain unreported. The following section summarizes the main XO inhibitory peptides of marine origin. Table 8.2 details enzymatic digestion methods and inhibitory effects for both mixed and single marine-derived XO inhibitory peptides. Li found that 25 mg/mL of bonito hydrolysates showed 65.5% inhibitory activity against XO [37]. Hu found 62.79% inhibitory activity against XO by 15 mg/mL of round scad protein hydrolysates [38].

To identify the primary active components within peptide mixtures, researchers typically isolate and purify mixed peptides, characterize them *via* mass spectrometry to obtain defined sequences, and evaluate synthesized versions for activity. Figure 8.3 outlines the general workflow for enzymatic digestion and purification of peptide inhibitors. Murota identified two shark fin cartilage-derived peptides (YLDNY and SPPYWPY) lacking in vitro XO inhibitory activity. However, di/tripeptide fragments derived from YLDNY (e.g., Asp-Asn) exhibited XO inhibitory. The authors suggest bioactive fragments generated during digestion or absorption may exert inhibition or modulate endogenous inhibitors. These fragments showed IC_{50} values 13–23 times higher than allopurinol [39]. Li utilized bonito surimi

Table 8.2 Comparison of activity of peptide inhibitors of xanthine oxidase

	Raw material	Enzymolysis enzymes	Polypeptide sequence	In vitro XO inhibitory activity/IC_{50} values	Allopurinol IC_{50} values	XO inhibition activity in vivo	References
Mixture	Bonito	Neutral protease	–	The XO inhibition activity of 25 mg/mL of bonito hydrolysates was 65.5%	–	–	[37]
	Round scad	Neutral protease	–	The inhibitory activity of 15 mg/mL Round scad protein hydrolysates on XO was 62.79%	–	–	[38]
Single peptide inhibitors	Shark cartilage	Alkali protease	YLDNY	No activity in vitro	3.8×10^{-2} mmol/L	Hyperuricemia rat model: oral administration has anti-hyperuricemia activity, and intravenous injection of 5 mg/kg body weight can reduce serum uric acid levels	[39]
	Shark cartilage	Alkali protease	SPPYWPY	–	–	Hyperuricemia rat model: intravenous injection of 5 mg/kg body weight can reduce serum uric acid levels	[39]
	Bonito	Papain	PGACSN	–	–	Hyperuricemia rat model: rats treated with bonito hydrolysates had significantly lower serum uric acid levels	[37]
	Bonito	Papain	WML	The XO inhibitory activity of 20 mM WML was comparable to that of 20 μM allopurinol	–	Hyperuricemia rat model: rats treated with bonito hydrolysates had significantly lower serum uric acid levels	[37]
	Tuna	Alkali protease	FH	25.7 mM	0.022 mM	Hyperuricemic rat model: tuna protein hydrolysates can reduce serum and liver XO activities in hyperuricemic rats	[40]
	Skipjack tuna	Neutral protease	ACECD	7.23 mg/mL	–	–	[41]
	Tuna protein	Pepsin, trypsin, and chymotrypsin	EEAK	173.00 ± 0.06 μM	–	–	[42]
	Round scad	Neutral protease	FPSV	22.61 ± 1.81% inhibition of FPSV at 5 mM	6.79 ± 0.25 μg/mL	–	[38]
	Round scad	Neutral protease	FPFP	20.09 ± 2.41% inhibition of FPFP at 5 mM	6.79 ± 0.25 μg/mL	–	[38]

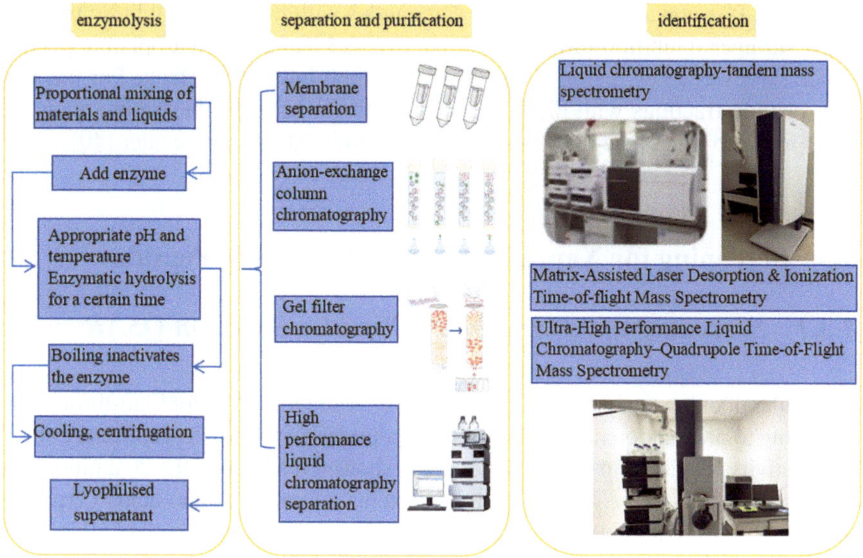

Fig. 8.3 Generic steps in the preparation of peptide inhibitors

protein digested with papain. Following ion-exchange and gel-filtration chromatography, they identified concentration-dependent inhibitory peptides PGACSN and WML *via* LC-ESI-MS/MS. [37] He hydrolyzed tuna protein with alkaline protease. Ethanol-soluble fractions were separated by Sephadex G-15 and HPLC, identifying 13 peptides. Among them, FH demonstrated the highest XO inhibitory activity with an IC_{50} value of 25.7 mM [40]. Zhong enzymatically digested skipjack tuna with neutral protease, isolating a 600–1000 Da fraction. After membrane separation, the pentapeptide ACECD was analyzed by MALDI-TOF/TOF-MS. The pentapeptide had strong XO inhibitory activity with an IC_{50} value of 7.23 mg/mL [41]. Yu identified the XO inhibitory tetrapeptide EEAK from tuna protein. EEAK had strong in vitro XO inhibitory activity with an IC_{50} value of 173.00 ± 0.06 μM [42]. Hu digested *Dosidicus gigas* with neutral protease. Isolation and purification were performed using immobilized metal affinity chromatography (IMAC). Four peptides were identified by nano-HPLC-MS/MS. Among them, both FPSV and FPFP had high XO inhibitory activities, with 22.61 ± 1.81% and 20.09 ± 2.41% inhibition at 5 mM, respectively [38].

Through comparative analysis of the identified peptide sequences, it is known that peptides with XO inhibitory activity have the following characteristics: (1) neutral or weakly basic peptides exhibit greater XO inhibitory than acidic peptides [37]. (2) Peptides that contain Trp exhibit relatively strong XO inhibitory activity, and the position of the Trp residue within these peptides also plays a role in determining their XO inhibitory potency. Notably, incorporating additional Trp residues effectively enhances the XO inhibitory activity of such peptides [43]. (3) Hu suggested that the substances that exert XO inhibitory activity in the enzymatic hydrolysate are mainly peptides of small molecules [38]. (4) Basic amino acids are critical for activity in Phe-containing dipeptides. Dipeptides with both Phe and basic residues show stronger inhibition [40]. (5) XO's active site features a hydrophobic pocket, which serves as a key region where XOI exert their inhibitory effects. For this reason, peptide fractions with higher concentrations of hydrophobic amino acids are more likely to access the hydrophobic region within XO's active center [40].

8.3 Screening for Xanthine Oxidase Inhibitory Peptides

8.3.1 Screening of XO Inhibitory Peptides Based on QSAR

Molecular docking analysis (Fig. 8.4) employed AutoDock Vina for high-throughput screening to predict potential XO inhibitory peptides and conduct preliminary structure–activity relationship studies. The results showed that among the 20 amino acids commonly found in the composition of proteins, aromatic amino acids (Trp, Tyr, Phe), especially Trp, had higher Vina scores. These residues effectively inhibit XO catalytic activity and are predicted to confer high inhibitory potency in peptides. The XO inhibitory activity of the polypeptides was influenced by the amino acid position. Overall, aromatic amino acid residues in the N-terminal position favored peptides with higher Vina scores and were able to exert higher XO inhibitory activity. The amino acid Trp acts on XO in a manner similar to allopurinol, capable of binding to key XO amino acid residues, including Glu802, Leu873, Ser876, Arg880, Phe914, Phe1009, Thr1010, Val1011, Leu1014, Ala1078, and Ala1079. This interaction induces a high Vina score in the peptide, enabling it to exert strong XO inhibitory activity [43]. Mao successfully and rapidly screened seven novel XO inhibitory peptides, YNITGW, GDEY, AGDY, PDARG, YGDE, VTGW, and EDDDA, from the whole protein sequences of the Pacific white shrimp, *Penaeus vannamei*, by molecular docking and BLAST techniques. It was found that increasing the number of Trp residues in the peptides could effectively enhance the XO inhibitory activity of the peptides and provide better inhibition of XO [44]. Bu combined bioinformatics prediction and analytical experiments to identify three new XO inhibitory peptides and explain their inhibitory mechanisms. ICRK, MMER, and FDAK peptides have some inhibitory effects and can be used as potential uric acid-lowering drugs [45].

8.3.2 Immobilized Enzyme Technology

Liu successfully synthesized silica-coated Fe_3O_4 nanoparticles immobilized with xanthine oxidase. The nanoparticles were characterized using Fourier transform infrared spectroscopy (FT-IR), X-ray powder diffraction (XRD), transmission

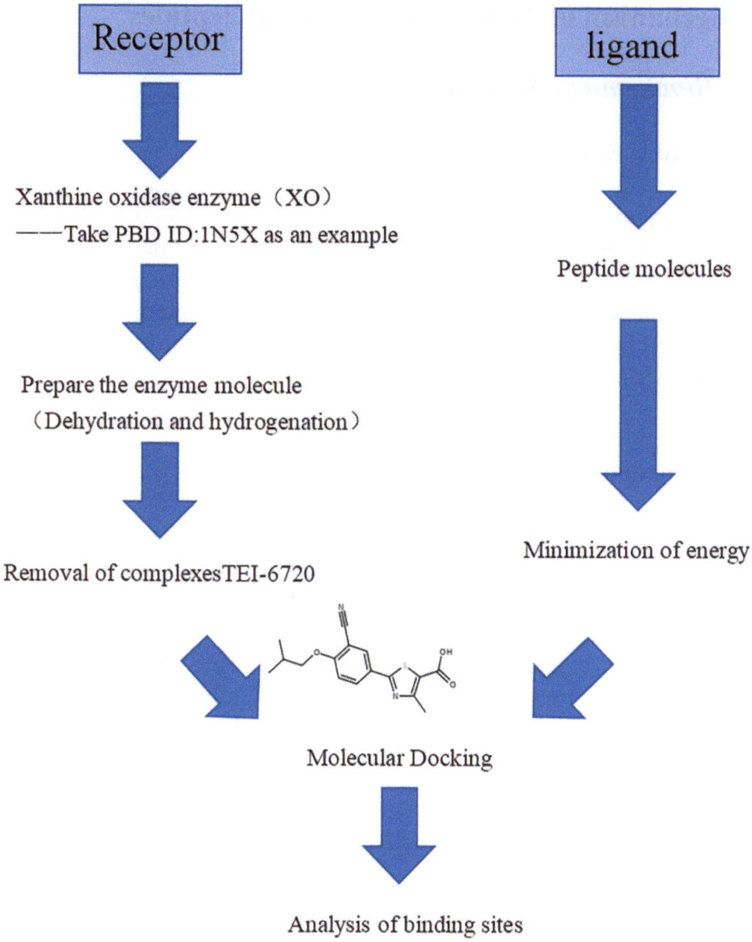

Fig. 8.4 Molecular docking flow chart

electron microscopy (TEM), and vibrating sample magnetometry (VSM). Researchers developed a method for screening inhibitors using these immobilized XO nanoparticles. When applied to Echinacea extracts, this method identified gardenin B and eupatorin as active compounds, with IC_{50} values of 1.488 ± 0.05 μg/mL and 11.197 ± 0.21 μg/mL, respectively [46].

Hu employed *Dosidicus gigas* as the starting material and generated hydrolysates using neutral protease. IMAC was employed for separation and purification. Four peptides were identified using nano-HPLC-MS/MS. Of these, peptides FPSV and FPFP exhibited potent XO inhibitory activity, with respective inhibition rates of 22.61 ± 1.81% and 20.09 ± 2.41% at a concentration of 5 mM [38].

8.4 Mechanism of Activity of Functional Peptides

8.4.1 Biochemical Methods

8.4.1.1 Double Enzyme Coupling Method

During the catalytic oxidation of xanthine, XO consumes 1 mol of molecular O_2 and 1 mol of H_2O per mole of xanthine oxidized, producing 1 mol of uric acid and 1 mol of H_2O_2. The resulting H_2O_2 is decomposed by horseradish peroxidase (HRP), enabling 4-aminoantipyrine and phenol to form a red quinoneimine dye. XO activity is quantified by spectrophotometrically measuring the absorbance of this chromogen in the visible spectrum [47].

8.4.1.2 Ultraviolet Spectrophotometry

XO catalyzes the oxidation of hypoxanthine and xanthine to uric acid, generating oxygen radicals. Consequently, inhibiting XO activity reduces uric acid levels. This mechanism enables the in vitro screening of XO inhibitors by quantifying their effect on enzyme activity. A common method quantifies XO activity by measuring uric acid absorbance at 290 nm using UV spectrophotometry. Absorbance is directly proportional to XO activity [48]. Alternatively, HPLC can quantify XO activity by measuring the uric acid peak area at 290 nm, where a larger peak area corresponds to higher activity.

8.4.2 Cell Model

Limited reports exist on using cellular models of hyperuricemia to screen for urate-lowering drugs. For example, Gao developed a hyperuricemia model using alpha mouse liver 12 (AML12) cells and human proximal tubular epithelial (HK-2) cells. They used adenosine and xanthine to induce hyperuricemia in an in vitro cell model. The xanthine oxidase inhibitor N-(9,10-anthraquinone-2-ylcarbonyl) (NAY) significantly inhibited XO activity and reduced uric acid levels in this model [49].

8.4.3 Animal Model

Animal models of hyperuricemia are typically established through three primary methods: (1) eating uric acid, high-purine foods, or uric acid precursors directly can raise xanthine oxidase activity. This boosts uric acid production, creating a hyperuricemia model. (2) Using drugs to block uric acid excretion can increase blood uric acid levels, leading to hyperuricemia. Common drugs for this include adenine and niacin. (3) Uricase inhibition. Uricase normally catalyzes urate oxidation to allantoin; thus, its inhibition elevates serum urate levels. Potassium oxonate (PO) is a commonly used uricase inhibitor. Elevated serum urate levels strongly correlate with kidney disease progression, systemic inflammation, and organ dysfunction. These levels also sensitively correspond to clinical and laboratory parameters such as blood urea nitrogen (BUN) and serum creatinine (SCR). Notably, SCR is a more specific renal function indicator than BUN [50].

Li established a hyperuricemia rat model using PO. Serum urate (SUA) levels were quantified using phosphotungstic acid assays, BUN and SCR levels were determined using commercial kits, while kidney histopathology was assessed *via* hematoxylin–eosin (HE) staining. Results demonstrated that bonito hydrolysate (BH) exhibited significant anti-hyperuricemia activity during chronic administration. Histopathological analysis confirmed BH attenuated renal damage in hyperuricemia rats [37]. Similarly, Murata employed PO to establish a hyperuricemia rat model. Their results indicated shark cartilage aqueous extract significantly reduced urate levels. Intravenous injection (5 mg/kg) of peptides YLDNY and SPPYWPY demonstrated significant anti-hyperuricemia activity, though neither exhibited XOI in vitro. In contrast, some dipeptides or tripeptides derived from these small-molecule peptides such as Asp-Asn, Leu-Asp-Asn, Asp-Asn-Tyr, Leu-Asp-Asn-Tyr showed in vitro XO inhibitory activity. This may be due to the fact that YLDNY and others are broken down into smaller peptides during digestion and absorption, thus exerting XO inhibitory activity or inducing endogenous XO inhibitory activity [39]. He similarly confirmed tuna protein hydrolysate's anti-hyperuricemia effects using PO-induced hyperuricemia rats [40]. The effects of uric acid-lowering peptides are usually tested using animal models of hyperuricemia, and the in vivo uric acid-lowering effect is evaluated using SUA, BUN, SCR levels, renal tissue sections, and mRNA expression of ADA and XO.

8.4.4 Molecular Docking

Molecular docking is commonly used to elucidate mechanisms of xanthine oxidase XO inhibition by peptides. The molybdenum pterin center, which incorporates Mo-pt, serves as a crucial site for XO catalysis. It is linked to the pterin through two S atoms, forming a tetrahedral structure with the O in Mo=O serving as the apex. Key catalytic residues include Glu802, Arg880, and Glu1261 (bovine XO numbering) [51]. WPPKN occupies the hydrophobic channel, sterically hindering xanthine binding to XO. Conversely, ADIYTE binds surface residues on the B-chain, obstructing substrate access to the channel. ADIYTE exhibits weaker XO inhibition than WPPKN due to suboptimal interactions with the molybdenum-binding domain [50]. Li molecularly docked 20 amino acids, 400 dipeptides and 8000 tripeptides. The results indicate that Trp demonstrated mixed-type inhibition, forming interactions with catalytic residues including Glu802, Arg880, Phe914, and the molybdenum center (Mo3004), *via* hydrogen bonding, hydrophobic contacts, and van der Waals forces—similar to allopurinol's binding mode. PPKNW is a noncompetitive inhibitory type, and PPKNW interacts with residues Phe649, Leu712, His875, Glu879, Phe883, Pro1012, Phe1013, Tyr1140, Phe1142, and Glu1143, including hydrogen-bonding, hydrophobic, and van der Waals interactions. WDQW is a mixed type of inhibition type, and WDQW interacts with key residues Glu802, Leu873, Ser876, Arg880, Phe914, Phe1009, Thr1010, Val1011, Leu1014, Ala1078, Ala1079, and Mos3004 [43]. Hydrogen bonds and attractive charges exist between the amino acid residues of PGACSN and the key residues of XO, Glu802, Arg880, and Glu1261. WML, on the other hand, enters the hydrophobic channel mainly through hydrophobic interactions, and then only one hydrogen bond (2.036 Å) is observed between Leu and Asn768, and a π-sulfur bond is formed between Trp and the Mos3004 active site [37]. FH has two hydrogen bonds with Ser876 and Thr1010 in XO and a π-π stacking interaction with Phe914 [40]. The entire sequence of IIAPPER could not be docked successfully, while the sequences IIAPPE and IAPPER after removing any 1 amino acid from both ends could be docked successfully. Since the xanthine oxidase active pocket is near the surface of the protein and not inside, it is therefore reasonable to speculate that the active peptide does not enter the active pocket completely, but that some of it remains on the outside of the active pocket, preventing the substrate from entering the active center. The same effect of inhibiting enzyme activity was achieved [44]. ACECD inserts into the Mo-atom-containing active center of XO and interacts with amino acid residues around the active center through hydrogen bonding, hydrophobic and van der Waals forces, etc. There may be competition for the same binding site between ACECD and the substrate xanthine [41].

8.5 Summary

Marine shellfish meat is rich, tender, delicious, high in protein, and nutrient dense. Research advances have also been made in identifying uric acid-lowering peptides from marine shellfish. However, protein-derived small-molecule uric acid-lowering peptides have garnered significant research interest due to their low preparation cost, safety, ease of absorption, high activity, stability, and specificity. A variety of bioactive peptides isolated from marine shellfish have demonstrated efficacy in promoting bone health, lowering blood pressure, reducing blood clot formation, among other functions. The field of uric acid-lowering peptides is emerging, with such peptides already identified in various marine fish species. It is anticipated that uric acid-lowering peptides derived from marine shellfish will be discovered in the coming years.

The meat of Marine shellfish is fat and tender, delicious, high protein content, and rich in nutrients. There are also research advances in marine shellfish uric acid-lowering peptides. However, protein-derived small-molecule uric acid-lowering peptides have attracted the attention of researchers because of their low preparation cost, safety, easy absorption, high activity, stability, and specificity. A variety of active peptides have been found in marine shellfish, which have made some progress in bone promotion, lowering blood pressure, lowering blood clots, and so on. The field of uric acid-lowering peptides has just begun, and uric acid-lowering peptides have been found in a variety of marine fish. It is believed that uric acid-lowering peptides from marine shellfish will also be discovered soon.

References

1. Zhou X, Liu K, Shi C, Zhang M, Liu S, Hou C, Di B. Estimation of the spatial pattern of gout prevalence across China by wastewater-based epidemiology. Sci Total Environ. 2024;924:171565.
2. Dehlin M, Jacobsson L, Roddy E. Global epidemiology of gout: prevalence, incidence, treatment patterns and risk factors. Nat Rev Rheumatol. 2020;16(7):380–90.
3. Mattiuzzi C, Lippi G. Recent updates on worldwide gout epidemiology. Clin Rheumatol. 2020;39(4):1061–3.
4. Choi HK, Niu J, Neogi T, Chen CA, Chaisson C, Hunter D, Zhang Y. Nocturnal risk of gout attacks. Arthritis Rheumatol. 2015;67(2):555–62.
5. Kuo CF, Grainge MJ, Zhang W, Doherty M. Global epidemiology of gout: prevalence, incidence and risk factors. Nat Rev Rheumatol. 2015;11(11):649–62.
6. Robinson PC. Gout – an update of aetiology, genetics, co-morbidities and management. Maturitas. 2018;118:67–73.
7. Mitchell S, Manounah L, Liedgens H, Johannes E. The effect of serum uric acid levels on tophus status and flares in patients with gout: a systematic review. Ann Rheum Dis. 2017;76(S2):1369–70.
8. Dalbeth N, Choi HK, Joosten LAB, Khanna PP, Matsuo H, Perez-Ruiz F, Stamp LK. Gout. Nat Rev Rheumatol. 2019;5(1):69.
9. Li H, Zhao M, Su G, Lin L, Wang Y. Effect of soy sauce on serum uric acid levels in hyperuricemic rats and identification of flazin as a potent xanthine oxidase inhibitor. J Agric Food Chem. 2016;64(23):4725–34.
10. Zhang S, Li D, Fan M, Yuan J, Xie C, Yuan H, Xie H, Gao H. Mechanism of reactive oxygen species-guided immune responses in gouty arthritis and potential therapeutic targets. Biomolecules. 2024;14(8):978.
11. Drug and Therapeutics Bulletin. Latest guidance on the management of gout. Br Med J. 2018;362:k2893.
12. Yin H, Liu N, Chen J. The role of the intestine in the development of hyperuricemia. Front Immunol. 2022;13:845684.
13. Lin P, Chen Z, Lin J. Therapeutic drugs of gout: the progress in target selection. Int J Rheum Dis. 2024;27(1):e15022.
14. Petru L, Pavelcova K, Sebesta I, Stiburkova B. Genetic background of uric acid metabolism in a patient with severe chronic tophaceous gout. Clin Chim Acta. 2016;460:46–9.
15. Tai V, Merriman TR, Dalbeth N. Genetic advances in gout: potential applications in clinical practice. Curr Opin Rheumatol. 2019;31(2):144–51.
16. Choi HK, Mount DB, Reginato AM. Pathogenesis of gout. Ann Intern Med. 2005;143(7):499–516.
17. Roman YM. The Daniel K. Inouye College of Pharmacy Scripts: perspectives on the epidemiology of gout and hyperuricemia. Hawaii J Med Public Health. 2019;78(2):71–6.
18. Stamp LK, O'Donnell JL, Chapman PT. Emerging therapies in the long-term management of hyperuricaemia and gout. Intern Med J. 2007;37(4):258–66.

19. Zhao ZA, Jiang Y, Chen YY, Wu T, Lan QS, Li YM, Li L, Yang Y, Lin CT, Cao Y, Zhou PZ, Guo JY, Tian YX, Pang JX. CDER167, a dual inhibitor of URAT1 and GLUT9, is a novel and potent uricosuric candidate for the treatment of hyperuricemia. Acta Pharmacol Sin. 2022;43(1):121–32.
20. Boger WP, Strickland SC. Probenecid (benemid); its uses and side-effects in 2,502 patients. AMA Arch Intern Med. 1955;95(1):83–92.
21. Pui K, Gow PJ, Dalbeth N. Efficacy and tolerability of probenecid as urate-lowering therapy in gout; clinical experience in high-prevalence population. J Rheumatol. 2013;40(6):872–6.
22. Strilchuk L, Fogacci F, Cicero AF. Safety and tolerability of available urate-lowering drugs: a critical review. Expert Opin Drug Saf. 2019;18(4):261–71.
23. Kuzell WC, Glover RP, Gibbs JO, Blau RA. Effect of sulfinpyrazone on total serum cholesterol in gout: a long-term study. Am J Med Sci. 1964;248(2):164–74.
24. Bardin T, Richette P. Novel uricosurics. Rheumatology (Oxford). 2018;57(1):42–6.
25. Yashika G, Vishant G, Rajeshwari G, Shyam GR, Arun K. Lesinurad, a novel uricosuric drug for allopurinol-refractory gout patients. J Clin Diagn Res. 2018;12(2):1–5.
26. Sidari A, Hill E. Diagnosis and treatment of gout and pseudogout for everyday practice. Prim Care. 2018;45(2):213–36.
27. Rheumatology AF, Rheumatologist PK. The management of gout. Aust Prescr. 2016;39(4):119–22.
28. Hosny NM, Atia NN, El-Gizawy SM. A review on: analysis of certain drugs used in gout treatment. Microchem J. 2019;149:149.
29. Robinson PC, Dalbeth N. Advances in pharmacotherapy for the treatment of gout. Expert Opin Pharmacother. 2015;16(4):533–46.
30. Thompson PL. Colchicine in cardiovascular disease: repurposing an ancient gout drug. Clin Ther. 2019;41(1):8–10.
31. Sala A, Proschak E, Steinhilber D, Rovati GE. Two-pronged approach to anti-inflammatory therapy through the modulation of the arachidonic acid cascade. Biochem Pharmacol. 2018;158:161–73.
32. Marouf R, Chtioui H, Girardin FR, Buclin T, Diezi L. Pharmacovigilance. Withdrawal and rebound effects: not just with psychotropic drugs. Rev Med Suisse. 2024;20(856–7):96–101.
33. Shannon JA, Cole SW. Pegloticase: a novel agent for treatment-refractory gout. Ann Pharmacother. 2012;46(3):368–76.
34. Nyborg A, Ward C, Zacco A, Chacko B, Grinberg L, Geoghegan JC, Bean R, Wendeler M, Bartnik F, O'Connor E, Gruia F, Iyer V, Feng H, Roy V, Berge M, Miner JN, Wilson DM, Zhou D, Nicholson S, Wilker C, Wu CY, Wilson S, Jermutus L, Wu H, Owen DA, Osbourn J, Coats S, Baca M. A therapeutic uricase with reduced immunogenicity risk and improved development properties. PLoS One. 2016;11(12):e0167935.
35. Cammalleri L, Malaguarnera M. Rasburicase represents a new tool for hyperuricemia in tumor lysis syndrome and in gout. Int J Med Sci. 2007;4(2):83–93.
36. Yu D, Du J, He P, Wang N, Li L, Liu Y, Yang C, Xu H, Li Y. Identification of natural xanthine oxidase inhibitors: virtual screening, anti-xanthine oxidase activity, and interaction mechanism. Int J Biol Macromol. 2024;259(Pt 2):129286.
37. Li Y, Kang X, Li Q, Shi C, Lian Y, Yuan E, Zhou M, Ren J. Anti-hyperuricemic peptides derived from bonito hydrolysates based on *in vivo* hyperuricemic model and *in vitro* xanthine oxidase inhibitory activity. Peptides. 2018;107:45–53.
38. Hu X, Zhou Y, Zhou S, Chen S, Wu Y, Li L, Yang X. Purification and identification of novel xanthine oxidase inhibitory peptides derived from round scad (*Decapterus maruadsi*) protein hydrolysates. Mar Drugs. 2021;19(10):538.
39. Murota I, Taguchi S, Sato N, Park EY, Nakamura Y, Sato K. Identification of antihyperuricemic peptides in the proteolytic digest of shark cartilage water extract using *in vivo* activity-guided fractionation. J Agric Food Chem. 2014;62(11):2392–7.
40. He W, Su G, Sun-Waterhouse D, Waterhouse GIN, Zhao M, Liu Y. In vivo anti-hyperuricemic and xanthine oxidase inhibitory properties of tuna protein hydrolysates and its isolated fractions. Food Chem. 2019;272:453–61.

41. Zhong H, Abdullah, Zhang Y, Deng L, Zhao M, Tang J, Zhang H, Feng F, Wang J. Exploring the potential of novel xanthine oxidase inhibitory peptide (ACECD) derived from Skipjack tuna hydrolysates using affinity-ultrafiltration coupled with HPLC-MALDI-TOF/TOF-MS. Food Chem. 2021;347:1–9.
42. Yu Z, Kan R, Wu S, Guo H, Zhao W, Ding L, Zheng F, Liu J. Xanthine oxidase inhibitory peptides derived from tuna protein: virtual screening, inhibitory activity, and molecular mechanisms. J Sci Food Agric. 2021;101(4):1349–54.
43. Li Q, Shi C, Wang M, Zhou M, Liang M, Zhang T, Yuan E, Wang Z, Yao M, Ren J. Tryptophan residue enhances *in vitro* walnut protein-derived peptides exerting xanthine oxidase inhibition and antioxidant activities. J Funct Foods. 2019;53:276–85.
44. Mao Z, Jiang H, Sun J, Mao X. Virtual screening and structure optimization of xanthine oxidase inhibitory peptides from whole protein sequences of Pacific white shrimp *via* molecular docking. Food Chem. 2023;429:136837.
45. Bu Y, Wang F, Zhu W, Li X. Combining bioinformatic prediction and assay experiment to identify novel xanthine oxidase inhibitory peptides from Pacific bluefin tuna (*Thunnus Orientalis*). E3S Web Conf. 2020;185:1–5.
46. Liu L, Yuan M, Huang S, Li J, Li D, Zhao L. Analysis of xanthine oxidase inhibitors from Clerodendranthus spicatus with xanthine oxidase immobilized silica coated Fe_3O_4 nanoparticles. Appl Sci. 2018;8(2):158.
47. Schmidt HM, Kelley EE, Straub AC. The impact of xanthine oxidase (XO) on hemolytic diseases. Redox Biol. 2019;21:101072.
48. Yasmineh WG. Simple ultraviolet spectrophotometric method for the determination of serum guanase activity. Clin Biochem. 1988;21(4):239–43.
49. Gao T, Xu J, Xiao Y, Li J, Hu W, Su X, Shen X, Yu W, Chen Z, Huang B, Li H, Wang X. Therapeutic effects and mechanisms of N-(9,10-anthraquinone-2-ylcarbonyl) xanthine oxidase inhibitors on hyperuricemia. Front Pharmacol. 2022;13:950699.
50. Li Q, Kang X, Shi C, Li Y, Majumder K, Ning Z, Ren J. Moderation of hyperuricemia in rats *via* consuming walnut protein hydrolysate diet and identification of new antihyperuricemic peptides. Food Funct. 2018;9(1):107–16.
51. White WB. Gout, xanthine oxidase inhibition, and cardiovascular outcomes. Circulation. 2018;138(11):1127–9.

Chapter 9
Marine Shellfish Protein and Taste Peptides

Ming Du, Shaoyun Wang, Maolin Tu, and Baifeng Fu

Abstract This chapter synthesizes recent advances in marine shellfish protein research, focusing particularly on umami peptides derived from these proteins. First, it highlights the fundamental role of umami taste perception mediated by its specific receptors. Next, the chapter systematically reviews the classification and signaling mechanisms of umami receptors. Subsequently, it explores umami peptide production methods, including enzymatic hydrolysis, chemical synthesis, enzymatic approaches, biotechnological production, and microbial fermentation, and evaluates analytical characterization techniques, such as sensory evaluation by trained panels and electronic tongue analysis. Finally, it examines the structure–activity relationships of umami peptides, analyzing key structural determinants, including molecular weight, amino acid composition, and sequence configuration. The chapter concludes with an exploration of AI-driven approaches for accelerating umami peptide discovery and development.

Keywords Marine shellfish protein · Taste peptide · Umami · Receptor · Preparation

Sour, sweet, bitter, umami, and salty represent the five fundamental taste modalities in human sensory perception. Advances in bioactive peptide research reveal that these functional molecules can elicit multiple taste sensations, driving increased discovery of taste-specific peptides for each modality. Marine-derived seafood is particularly valued for its distinct salty and umami profiles, with shellfish-derived

M. Du (✉)
College of Food Science and Engineering, Dalian Ocean University, Dalian, China

S. Wang
Biological Science and Engineering, Fuzhou University, Fuzhou, China

M. Tu
Food Science and Engineering, Ningbo University, Ningbo, China

B. Fu
Food Science and Engineering, Dalian Polytechnic University, Dalian, China

M. Du, S. Cheng (eds.), *Bioactive Proteins and Peptides from Marine Shellfish*,
https://doi.org/10.1007/978-981-95-3937-6_9

taste peptides predominantly associated with these two taste qualities. Umami peptides enhance savory perception while maintaining flavor palatability during salt and sugar reduction—a critical attribute for low-sodium dietary needs [1]. Conversely, salty peptide research remains limited, partly due to cost constraints. These dipeptides often exhibit concomitant umami or sour notes [2]. Consequently, this chapter focuses specifically on umami taste mechanisms and umami peptides.

9.1 Taste and Taste Receptors

Taste perception constitutes a critical physiological system in humans. Scientific evidence establishes that distinct taste modalities are mediated by specific bioactive compounds essential for physiological functions [3]. Sweet peptides, exhibiting sweetness intensities up to 150-fold higher than sucrose, are increasingly identified in plant extracts. Salty peptides (predominantly dipeptides) occur less frequently and may impart concomitant sour or umami sensations. There is relatively little research on acidic peptides, often considered part of umami peptides, with representative substances including γ-glutamyl peptides such as Glu-γ-Gly, Glu-γ-Ala, Glu-γ-Glu, and γ-Glu-Tyr. Since bitterness is not favored by people, bitter peptides are rarely used in taste research, but studies by Pripp [4] and Upadhyaya [5] have found that bitter peptides possess blood pressure-lowering activity.

Marine shellfish products are generally loved for their delicious and moderately salty taste. Enzymatic hydrolysis of shellfish releases umami compounds employed in seasoning development to amplify both umami and salty perception. Umami denotes the characteristic savory taste exemplified by monosodium glutamate (MSG) and certain amino acids [6]. Umami substances are typically divided into five major categories: free amino acids (including glutamic acid and aspartic acid), nucleotides and their salts (including 5′-inosinic acid, 5′-guanylic acid, and 5′-adenylic acid), organic acids and their salts (including succinic acid and sodium succinate), organic bases (including betaine and trimethylamine N-oxide), and umami peptides. Umami peptides are defined as umami-imparting sequences either isolated from food sources or synthetically produced. Taste perception occurs not only orally but also *via* gastrointestinal tract receptors. This perception can affect the secretion of hormones in the body, as well as the absorption and utilization of sugars [7]. Consequently, umami peptide extraction from marine shellfish holds considerable promise for flavor enhancement.

9.1.1 Umami Taste Transduction Mechanisms

In the process of umami perception, it is generally believed that umami substances first pass through the small openings (taste pores) on the base of the taste buds on the tongue, then specifically bind to umami receptors. Triggering intracellular signaling cascades that generate synaptic transmission conveying savory perception to cortical centers (Fig. 9.1) [8–10].

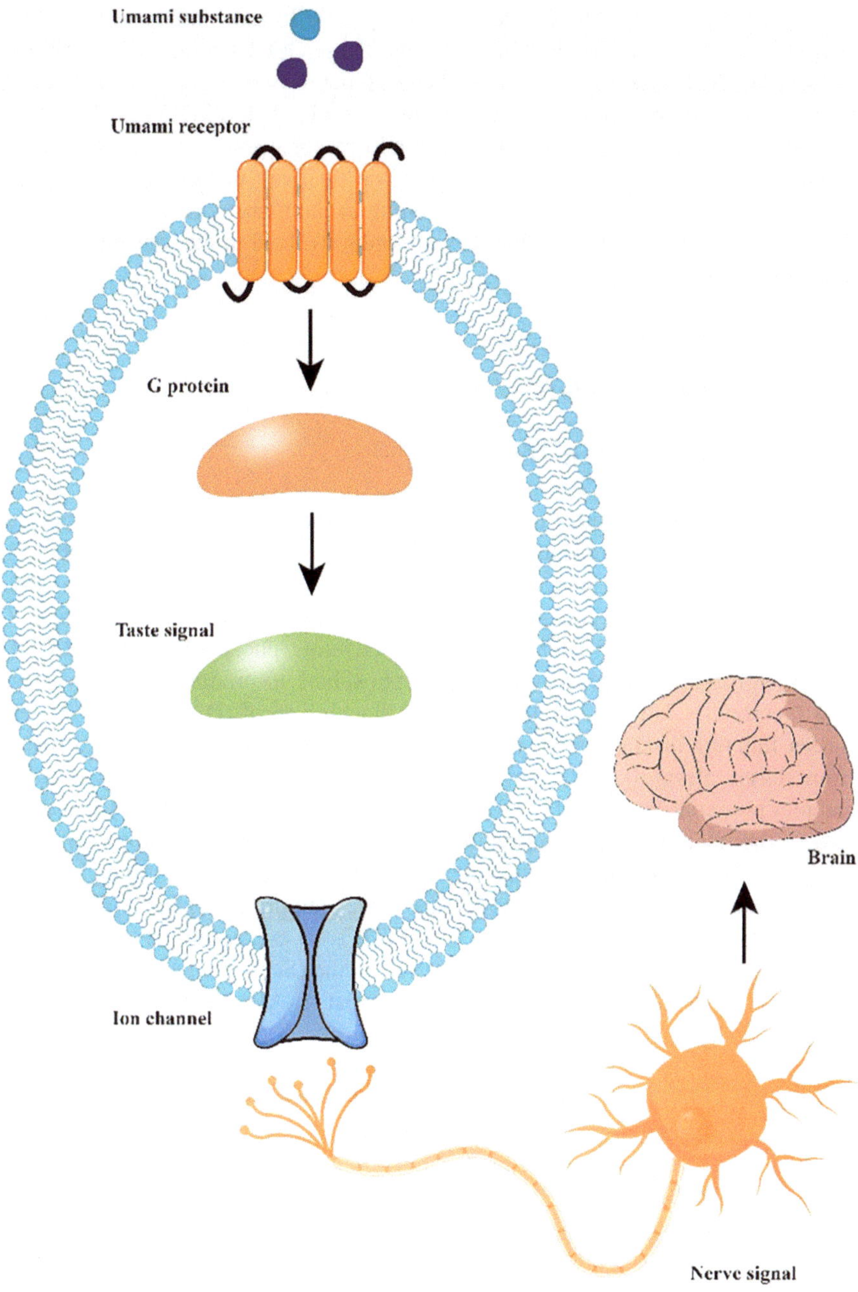

Fig. 9.1 Schematic diagram of umami signal transmission and neural signal transduction in taste cells

Umami perception critically depends on specific ligand binding to G protein-coupled receptors (GPCRs) within taste buds. These GPCRs comprise two primary classes. The first class, the T1R1/T1R3 heterodimer, serves as the canonical umami receptor recognizing diverse L-amino acids. Notably, T1R1/T1R3 knockout mice exhibit abolished umami preference but retain responsiveness, indicating parallel receptor pathways [11–13]. The second class involves metabotropic glutamate receptors (mGluR1 and mGluR4), functioning as auxiliary umami receptors [14]. Some researchers also believe that they are only involved in the transmission process of umami signals [15].

9.1.2 *Umami Receptors*

9.1.2.1 Heterodimer T1R1/T1R3

T1R1/T1R3 receptors detect umami-inducing amino acids, peptides, and nucleotides. The T1R1/T1R3 receptor is primarily expressed in type II cells within the fungiform papillae taste buds located on the anterior part of the tongue. It can bind with umami molecules, activating α-gustducin, causing the dissociation of the G protein's Gβ3 and Gγ13 subunits, thereby activating phospholipase C (PLCβ2), which hydrolyzes phosphatidylinositol bisphosphate to produce second messengers inositol 1,4,5-trisphosphate (IP3) and diacylglycerol (DAG) (Fig. 9.2). The further function of DAG is not yet clear. IP3 binding to its receptors releases Ca^{2+} from stores, elevating cytosolic Ca^{2+} levels. This Ca^{2+} surge activates transient receptor potential channel M5 (TRPM5) channels, mediating Na^{+} influx that depolarizes the membrane, triggering action potentials and ATP exocytosis. The released ATP acts as a neurotransmitter and is transmitted to the purinergic receptors on nerve fibers through the membrane-associated protein channel (CALHM1) [9, 16]. Grace demonstrated that T1R1/T1R3 co-expression is essential for responses to umami stimuli, including MSG, serine (Ser), and the agonist L(+)-2-Amino-4-phosphonobutanoic acid, umami agonist (L-AP4.13) [13].

9.1.2.2 Metabotropic Glutamate Receptors mGluR1 and mGluR4

Metabotropic glutamate receptor mGluR4 was first discovered in the brain and later found in taste cells as a taste-type mGluR4. This receptor localizes predominantly to circumvallate and foliate papillae, specifically expressed in taste receptor cells (TRCs) [17]. Umami stimulants, mostly substances similar to L-glutamate, bind to mGluR4. Receptor activation stimulates α-gustducin, subsequently activating phosphodiesterases (PDE) to decrease intracellular cyclic adenosine monophosphate (cAMP) levels. Reduced cAMP relieves its inhibition of cyclic nucleotide-gated (CNG) channels, triggering Ca^{2+} release from intracellular stores. This calcium flux induces membrane depolarization and neurotransmitter release [16]. Notably,

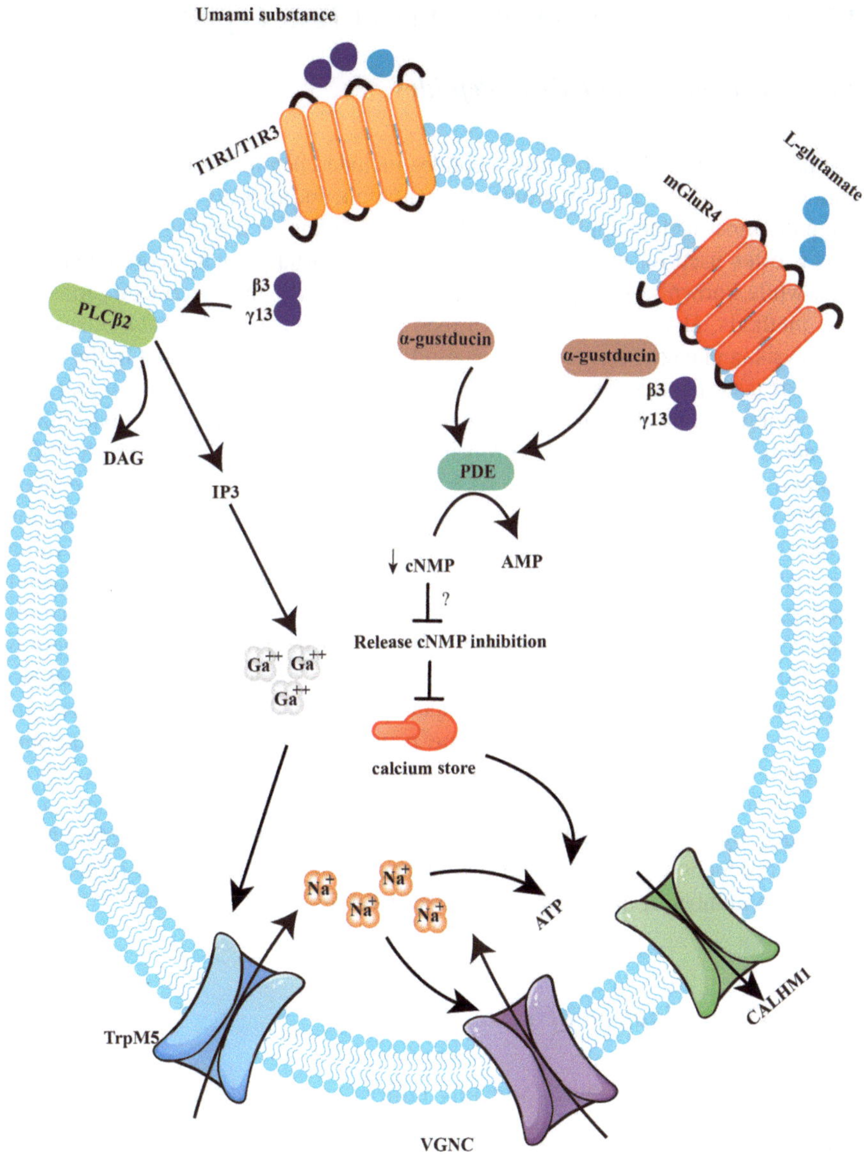

Fig. 9.2 Recognition and transduction of umami molecules on umami receptors T1R1/T1R3 and mGluR4

mGluR4 also exhibits sensitivity to nucleotides. Using RT-PCR and in situ hybridization, Nirupa demonstrated mGluR4 responsiveness to the MSG analog L-AP4, establishing it as a candidate umami receptor [18]. Complementarily, Keiko revealed mGluR4's functional role through knockout studies. mGluR4$^{-/-}$ mice exhibited diminished electrophysiological responses to glutamate and L-AP4 [15].

9.2 Preparation and Identification of Taste Peptides

9.2.1 Preparation of Taste Peptides

The preparation methods for taste peptides include chemical synthesis, enzymatic synthesis, bioengineering, microbial fermentation, and hydrolysis, with hydrolysis being the most widely applied method [19]. For unknown taste substances, hydrolysis is often used for preparation as it can yield substances with more intense flavors, while known taste peptides are more commonly synthesized using the other four methods. Hydrolysis can be further divided into acid hydrolysis, alkaline hydrolysis, and enzymatic hydrolysis. Acid hydrolysis is widely used in the preparation of taste peptides, with its advantages being high efficiency. However, it is challenging to control temperature and time. Moreover, it can produce toxic chloropropanols [20, 21]. Alkaline hydrolysis may cause racemization, which affects L-amino acids. Enzymatic hydrolysis is sensitive to pH, temperature, and enzyme dosage. Chemical synthesis and enzymatic synthesis methods follow the principle of base complementary pairing, utilizing amino acids and small peptides to synthesize taste peptides. Chemical synthesis is prone to racemization [19]. In bioengineering, the gene encoding a specific taste peptide is introduced into recipient cells, enabling the cells to produce the taste peptide. This method has the advantages of low cost and high yield, but the application process is hindered by the fact that bioengineering technology is not yet fully mature. Microbial fermentation involves the use of microorganisms to produce taste peptides under the action of microbial enzymes. However, the production effects can vary significantly depending on the strain of microorganism used. Traditional fermented condiments (e.g., soy sauce, fish sauce, oyster sauce, and Douban sauce) exemplify successful microbial flavor peptide production [22–24]. With the advancement of taste peptide research, an increasing number of marine flavor peptides have also been identified.

9.2.2 Determination of Taste Peptides

Current taste peptide analysis primarily utilizes two complementary approaches: sensory evaluation and electronic tongue systems. Sensory evaluation carries inherent subjectivity due to panelist bias, potentially introducing assessment errors. While electronic tongues may not fully replicate human perception, they offer high reproducibility across replicate measurements. Consequently, these methods are frequently integrated to leverage their complementary strengths. In addition, detection methods, including biosensors and gold nanoparticle sensors, are also being developed and applied in the determination of taste peptides.

9.2.2.1 Sensory Evaluation of Taste Peptides

Sensory evaluation in the study of taste peptides can be used for four aspects. The first aspect is to evaluate the taste profile of the isolated, extracted, or synthesized taste peptides. The second aspect is to evaluate the taste threshold of the taste peptides. The third aspect is to assess the contribution of taste peptides to the overall flavor. The fourth aspect is to evaluate the taste enhancement effect of taste peptides. These four aspects often assist each other and can be used for a comprehensive evaluation of taste peptides. Zhang applied this framework to Philippine clam peptides, evaluating taste profiles, detection thresholds, flavor contributions, and umami-enhancement effects [25]. When assessing the taste profile of taste peptides, standard samples representing the five basic tastes—sweet, bitter, sour, salty, and umami—are first selected. Then, the reconstituted taste peptides are scored on a scale, either a five-point or ten-point system. To evaluate the taste threshold of taste peptides, the three-point method is employed, in which the reconstituted solution is continuously diluted, and the assessor's perception of three samples (two of tap water and one of the reconstituted solution) is recorded. When the sensory panelists are unable to distinguish between the three solutions, the concentration of the reconstituted solution at that point is noted; and considered the taste threshold. Assessing the contribution of taste peptides to the overall flavor and their taste enhancement effects is done using taste dilution analysis methods. One such method is the taste dilution analysis (TDA), which records the dilution factor at the threshold measurement as the taste dilution (TD) value. First, the taste activity value (TAV) is calculated—the ratio of the concentration of a taste compound itself to the taste threshold detected by sensory methods. Then, the total contribution rate (%) is calculated as (TAV/Total TD Dilution Value) × 100. When the TAV of a single component is ≥1, it can be considered that this substance contributes to the taste. However, in complex systems, various taste components interact with each other. When the TAV is ≥0.1, it may also play a role in auxiliary taste enhancement. Another method is the comparative taste dilution analysis (cTDA). The calculation formula for cTDA differs from the TAV calculation formula in the way the TD value is determined. In cTDA, the TD value calculation involves dividing the sample into two identical parts, referred to as Part A and Part B. Part A follows the same method as described above, while Part B involves dissolving the sample in a solution of a taste standard with a low concentration. The three-point method is used to determine the TD value by comparing the TD values of each sample in Parts A and B. The sample that has a small TD value in Part A and a large TD value in Part B is identified as having a strong taste enhancement effect. For the determination of the taste enhancement coefficient, a standard solution with a certain concentration of the sample is prepared and then gradually diluted. Evaluators are asked to select the sample that has the same taste intensity as the standard. The taste enhancement coefficient is calculated as: $f = C1 / C2$. Here, $C1$ is the concentration of the standard, and $C2$ is the concentration of the mixed solution [26].

9.2.2.2 Electronic Tongue Evaluation of Taste Peptides

Instrumental analysis, particularly with an electronic tongue, primarily determines the taste profile of samples by using biosensor arrays with specific bioelectronic membranes. Additionally, similarity analysis of the collected multidimensional data is performed using the system's PCA capabilities [26]. Zhang further demonstrated that an electronic tongue can effectively evaluate the taste of hydrolyzed peanut meal products, finding a strong correlation between its analysis and sensory evaluation data [25].

9.2.2.3 Other Methods for Evaluating Taste Peptides

In recent years, research efforts have focused on developing methods for the more efficient, accurate, and rapid detection and screening of taste-active substances. Numerous new sensors have been invented, including biosensors and biomimetic nanosensors. The sensors currently in development still face challenges such as low stability, poor specificity for certain substances, and low sensitivity. Consequently, the screening and quantification of taste-active substances remains a significant challenge. Fan divided rabbit tongues into nine regions and immobilized taste bud tissue on the surface of glassy carbon electrodes to construct a taste bud biosensor. Their research revealed that the umami signal receptors T1R1/T1R3 are predominantly expressed in taste receptor cells at the tongue tip [27]. Li utilized the "Venus flytrap domain (VFTD)" of the human umami receptor subunit T1R1 to build a bionic conical nanochannel system. In this system, the passage of mixtures through the nanochannels triggers sensitive changes in transmembrane ionic flux, enabling the precise screening of umami substances [28]. Ahn extracted nanovesicles containing umami receptors (T1R1/T1R3) and sweet receptors (T1R2/T1R3) from human embryonic kidney (HEK-293) cells and immobilized these vesicles onto graphene surfaces to create a dual biosensor capable of simultaneously detecting both umami and sweet substances [29].

9.2.3 Taste Peptides and Their Umami Receptors

Marine-derived taste peptides typically exhibit an umami taste. Molecular docking simulates the interaction between umami peptides and the umami receptor T1R1/T1R3, providing a preliminary assessment of the peptides' umami taste potential. Scatchard analysis and molecular dynamics simulation are two primary methods used to analyze the binding interactions between ligands and receptors. Because the three-dimensional crystal structure and function of T1R1/T1R3 remain undetermined, homology modeling, often coupled with MD simulation, is commonly used to construct its three-dimensional structure. Homology modeling offers advantages such as lower computational requirements and high prediction accuracy. It is considered reasonable for protein three-dimensional structures when the homology reaches 30% [24]. The process of homologous modeling includes four parts: selecting an appropriate template from the Protein Data Bank (PDB), aligning and arranging the target and template protein sequences, constructing the conserved and flexible regions of the target protein model, and evaluating and optimizing the model structure through Ramachandran plots [30].

Molecular docking principles originate from the "lock and key" hypothesis, evolving into the induced fit theory. During docking simulations, the receptor's conformation undergoes adjustment to achieve optimal ligand binding. In their analysis of umami peptides from clams and mussels, Li [31] selected the amino acid sequences of the heterodimer T1R1/T1R3 from the UniProtKB database (https://www.uniprot.org/) and used the mGluR1 template (PDB ID: 1EWK) from the RCSB database (http://www.rcsb.org/). After analyzing seven peptide chains with Discovery Studio software, they found that all seven umami peptides bind to the receptor by inserting into the VFTD of the T1R3 subunit. This provides insights into the structural basis of umami perception by understanding the interaction between taste peptides and their receptors at the molecular level.

9.3 Structure–Activity Characteristics of Taste Peptides

The study of the structure–activity characteristics and the umami mechanism of umami peptides derived from marine shellfish has long been a subject of significant debate in academia. First, consensus is lacking regarding the specific molecular structures conferring umami taste—particularly the structure–umami taste correlation. Currently, research on the impact of peptide spatial conformation and amino acid configuration on umami taste has not reached a definitive conclusion [26]. Second, some umami peptides identified by previous researchers do not exhibit umami characteristics in subsequent measurements [32]. The octapeptide derived from beef was found to have not only umami but also sour and sweet tastes [33], whereas Van Wassenaar [34] and Tamura [35] upon synthesizing the same peptide and conducting taste tests, found no umami taste. Consequently, the taste mechanisms of umami peptides require further elucidation.

9.3.1 Molecular Weight Considerations

Peptides with a smaller molecular weight are generally capable of eliciting an umami taste. Umami peptides typically possess an amino acid backbone consisting of 3–9 carbon (C) atoms, with the most intense umami taste occurring when there are 4–6 C atoms. However, C can be substituted by oxygen (O), nitrogen (N), sulfur (S), or phosphorus (P). Using electronic tongue analysis, Li demonstrated that components less than 3 kDa in size from a *Meretrix lusoria* (clam) solution had a more umami taste profile compared to components greater than 3 kDa [31], which were closer to the taste of the original clam solution [25]. As the ultrafiltration time increased and the membrane flux continuously decreased, the umami taste significantly increased, while the fishy and bitter tastes noticeably diminished. A study has extracted 14 peptides from the Philippines clams, with molecular weights ranging between 491 and 945 Da. Among these, the peptide with the lowest umami threshold, KN-5, has a molecular weight of 547 Da. Molecular docking with T1R1/T1R3 revealed TD-8 and QK-8 as the lowest-energy binders to the T1R3 subunit. This suggests shorter peptides preferentially bind T1R3 to elicit umami taste. Conversely, Li reported no correlation between peptide length and binding energy to umami receptors [31]. The key amino acid residues involved in the binding of umami peptides to the umami receptor T1R1/T1R3 are Asp196, Glu128, His125, His368, Glu281, and Arg34. Some scholars believe that longer peptides are more easily perceived by umami receptors. On one hand, peptides of a certain length can shorten the docking distance with the umami receptors. On the other hand, longer peptide chains have greater flexibility in binding with umami receptors [24].

9.3.2 Amino Acid Composition

Different amino acids can exhibit distinct taste characteristics. Umami peptides frequently contain acidic residues glutamate (Glu) and aspartate (Asp) [24]. Sweet and salty tastes do not diminish with the addition of umami, they may be enhanced. In synthetic umami peptides, when salt or monosodium glutamate (MSG) is added, a synergistic effect occurs, resulting in an enhancement of both umami and salty tastes [36]. Spanier pioneered beef meat peptide (BMP) extraction from papain-hydrolyzed beef [37]. The amino acid composition of BMP is Lys-Gly-Asp-Glu-Glu-Ser-Leu-Ala, which includes both aspartic acid (Asp) and glutamic acid (Glu). Yamasaki identified the central Asp-Glu-Glu motif as responsible for BMP's acidic character [33]. However, the basic group at the N-terminus, composed of lysine (Lys) and glycine (Gly), mitigates the sourness of the acidic group. Although the C-terminal Ser-Leu-Ala is hydrophobic, N-terminal extension reduces overall hydrophobicity, enabling umami taste expression. Zhang extracted 14 novel umami peptides from the Philippines clams, with the sequences GRVSNCAA, SEEK, KEMQKN, KSAEN, QIEELEGK, TDVEQEGD, HNESQN, RGEPNND, TGDPEK, KGGGGP, TYLPVH, PAATIPE, GPAGPAGPR, and AGAGPTP [25]. The following is the ranking of the umami thresholds of the 14 umami peptide segments determined by sensory evaluation: KN-5 (0.23 mM) < QK-8 (0.27 mM) < GA-8 (0.32 mM) < KP-6 (0.53 mM) < HN-6 (0.69 mM) < AP-7 (0.88 mM) < TD-8 (1.12 mM) < GR-9 (1.28 mM) < KN-6 (1.29 mM) < PE-7 (1.43 mM) < SK-4 (2.03 mM) < RD-7 (2.50 mM) < TH-6 (2.74 mM) < TK-6 (3.10 mM), with KN-5 having the lowest threshold and QK-8 and GA-8 having the highest thresholds. The umami peptides can have lower thresholds because they contain not only acidic amino acids Asp and Glu but also basic amino acids and hydrophobic amino acids. The electronic tongue instrument was used to analyze the 14 peptide segments, with the scores from high to low, indicating AP-7 > QK-8 > KN-5 > KN-6 > KP-6 > SK-4 > HN-6 > PE-7 > TD-8 > GA-8 > GR-9 > RD-7 > TH-6 > TK-6. Although the scores from the electronic tongue analysis do not completely align with those from sensory evaluation, the overall trend is consistent. It is noted that some short peptides (QK-8, KN-5, KN-6, SK-4, HN-6, TD-8, RD-7, TK-6, and PE-7) do not contain the acidic amino acids Glu and Asp, yet they still exhibit umami taste. The umami taste of peptides is not only related to the types of amino acids they are composed of but also influenced by their spatial structure. Additionally, studies have shown that peptides containing Gly, Glu, and Gln residues demonstrate heightened umami potential [38, 39].

Li isolated seven novel umami peptides from enzymatically hydrolyzed *Meretrix lusoria* (clam) and *Meretrix petechialis* (blue clam) [31]. The sequences of these peptides were as follows: Gly-Leu-Leu-Pro-Asp-Gly-Thr-Pro-Arg, Arg-Pro-Asn-Pro-Phe-Glu-Asn-Arg, Ser-Thr-Met-Leu-Leu-Glu-Ser-Glu-Arg, Ala-Asn-Pro-Gly-Pro-Val-Arg-Asp-Leu-Arg, Gln-Val-Ala-Ile-Ala-His-Arg-Asp-Ala-Lys, Val-Leu-Pro-Thr-Asp-Gln-Asn-Phe-Ile-Leu-Arg, Val-Thr-Ala-Asp-Glu-Ser-Gln-Gln-Asp-Val-Leu-Lys. Subsequent synthesis of these seven umami peptides and sensory evaluation revealed that their taste thresholds were all 0.125 mg/mL, which is lower than that of MSG (0.3 mg/mL). The synthetic umami peptides were also described as having a softer and fuller flavor. Gly-Leu-Leu-Pro-Asp-Gly-Thr-Pro-Arg, Arg-Pro-Asn-Pro-Phe-Glu-Asn-Arg, and Ala-Asn-Pro-Gly-Pro-Val-Arg-Asp-Leu-Arg exhibited a distinct and prominent umami taste, along with a flavor-enhancing effect. Homology docking simulations confirmed successful binding to T1R1/T1R3. Analysis of their amino acid composition revealed the presence of at least one Asp and Glu in each peptide sequence. It indicates that the composition of amino acids influences the taste profile.

9.3.3 Sequence of Amino Acid

The sequence of amino acids can significantly influence the taste properties of peptides. Dipeptides with an acidic amino acid at the N-terminus and a hydrophilic or basic amino acid at the C-terminus typically have umami taste. If the order of the amino acids is reversed, the dipeptide may lose its taste characteristics [35, 40]. For instance, dipeptides such as Glu-Lys, Glu-Asp, Glu-Thr, Glu-Ser, and Glu-Glu exhibit umami taste, whereas their reversed counterparts lack this property. In longer umami peptides, however, this pattern is inverted. The N-terminus of BMP is a positively charged basic group, Lys-Gly-, closely followed by a negatively charged acidic group, -Asp-Glu-Glu-Glu-. And the hydrophobic group -Ser-Leu-Ala is located at its C-terminus [38]. Their synergistic action results in the umami taste of the BMP. Overall, it is necessary to have both hydrophobic, negatively charged, and positively charged groups to bind with the umami receptor and produce umami taste.

9.4 Summary

Marine shellfish represent rich sources of taste compounds and are processed into diverse seasonings and food products. This chapter primarily focuses on umami peptides found in marine shellfish. Firstly, umami is an essential taste in our perception of food, and its receptors play a crucial role in taste buds. Secondly, the chapter discusses the key technologies and processes involved in the production and preparation of umami peptides and analyzes their relationship with receptors. Finally, structural analysis of umami peptides establishes the foundation for efficient production and mechanistic understanding of their taste properties. Research on marine shellfish proteins and taste peptides enhances our understanding of their unique value in food development, offering valuable insights for advancing the food industry. At the same time, with the rapid development of artificial intelligence technology, its application in taste aspects of food is becoming increasingly widespread. AI-driven approaches show significant promise for accelerating the discovery of marine shellfish taste peptides.

References

1. Morita R, Ohta M, Hayabuchi H, Fujitani S, Tsuchihashi T. Quantitative verification of the effect of using an umami substance (L-glutamate) to reduce salt intake. Hypertens Res. 2020;43(6):579–81.
2. Gao T, Huang X, Chen X, Cai X, Huang J, Vincent G, Wang S. Advances in flavor peptides with sodium-reducing ability: a review. Crit Rev Food Sci Nutr. 2024;64(26):9568–84.
3. Temussi PA. The good taste of peptides. J Pept Sci. 2012;18(2):73–82.
4. Pripp AH, Ardoe Y. Modelling relationship between angiotensin-(I)-converting enzyme inhibition and the bitter taste of peptides. Food Chem. 2007;102(3):880–8.
5. Upadhyaya J, Pydi SP, Singh N, Aluko RE, Chelikani P. Bitter taste receptor T2R1 is activated by dipeptides and tripeptides. Biochem Biophys Res Commun. 2010;398(2):331–5.
6. Kurihara K. Umami the fifth basic taste: history of studies on receptor mechanisms and role as a food flavor. Biomed Res Int. 2015;2015:189402.
7. Gao J, Zhang S, Deng P, Wu Z, Lemaitre B, Zhai Z, Guo Z. Dietary L-Glu sensing by enteroendocrine cells adjusts food intake *via* modulating gut PYY/NPF secretion. Nat Commun. 2024;15(1):3514.
8. Cygankiewicz AI, Maslowska A, Krajewska WM. Molecular basis of taste sense: involvement of GPCR receptors. Crit Rev Food Sci Nutr. 2014;54(6):771–80.
9. Kinnamon S. Taste receptor signalling from tongues to lungs. Acta Physiol. 2012;204(2):158–68.
10. Xiao Y, Zhou H, Jiang L, Liu R, Chen Q. Epigenetic regulation of ion channels in the sense of taste. Pharmacol Res. 2021;172:105760.
11. Damak S, Rong M, Yasumatsu K, Kokrashvili Z, Varadarajan V, Zou S, Jiang P, Ninomiya Y, Margolskee RF. Detection of sweet and umami taste in the absence of taste receptor T1r3. Science. 2003;301(5634):850–3.
12. Li X, Staszewski L, Xu H, Durick K, Zoller M, Adler E. Human receptors for sweet and umami taste. Proc Natl Acad Sci USA. 2002;99(7):4692–6.
13. Zhao G, Zhang Y, Hoon M, Chandrashekar J, Erlenbach I, Ryba N, Zuker C. The receptors for mammalian sweet and umami taste. Cell. 2003;115(3):255–66.

14. Kunishima N, Shimada Y, Tsuji Y, Sato T, Yamamoto M, Kumasaka T, Nakanishi S, Jingami H, Morikawa K. Structural basis of glutamate recognition by a dimeric metabotropic glutamate receptor. Nature. 2000;407(6807):971–7.
15. Yasumatsu K, Manabe T, Yoshida R, Iwatsuki K, Uneyama H, Takahashi I, Ninomiya Y. Involvement of multiple taste receptors in umami taste: analysis of gustatory nerve responses in metabotropic glutamate receptor 4 knockout mice. J Physiol. 2015;593(4):1021–34.
16. Gilbertson TA, Damak S, Margolskee RF. The molecular physiology of taste transduction. Curr Opin Neurobiol. 2000;10(4):519–27.
17. Chaudhari N, Yang H, Lamp C, Delay E, Cartford C, Than T, Roper S. The taste of monosodium glutamate: membrane receptors in taste buds. J Neurosci. 1996;16(12):3817–26.
18. Chaudhari N, Roper S. Molecular and physiological evidence for glutamate (umami) taste transduction *via* a G protein-coupled receptor. Ann N Y Acad Sci. 2010;855:398–406.
19. Zhao Y, Zhang M, Devahastin S, Liu Y. Progresses on processing methods of umami substances: a review. Trends Food Sci Technol. 2019;93:125–35.
20. Li W, Gu Z, Yang Y, Zhou S, Liu Y, Zhang J. Non-volatile taste components of several cultivated mushrooms. Food Chem. 2014;143:427–31.
21. Song S, Li S, Fan L, Hayat K, Xiao Z, Chen L, Tang Q. A novel method for beef bone protein extraction by lipase-pretreatment and its application in the Maillard reaction. Food Chem. 2016;208:81–8.
22. Zhuang M, Lin L, Zhao M, Dong Y, Sun-Waterhouse D, Chen H, Qiu C, Su G. Sequence, taste and umami-enhancing effect of the peptides separated from soy sauce. Food Chem. 2016;206:174–81.
23. Bu Y, Liu Y, Luan H, Zhu W, Li X, Li J. Characterization and structure-activity relationship of novel umami peptides isolated from Thai fish sauce. Food Funct. 2021;12(11):5027–37.
24. Fu B, Wu D, Cheng S, Xu X, Zhang L, Wang L-S, El-Seedi H, Liu H, Du M. Three novel umami peptides derived from the alcohol extract of the Pacific oyster (*Crassostrea gigas*): identification, characterizations and interactions with T1R1/T1R3 taste receptors. Food Sci Human Wellness. 2023; 13(1):1–14.
25. Zhang Y, Gao X, Pan D, Zhang Z, Zhou T, Dang Y. Isolation, characterization and molecular docking of novel umami and umami-enhancing peptides from Ruditapes philippinarum. Food Chem. 2021;343:128522.
26. Qi L, Gao X, Pan D, Sun Y, Cai Z, Xiong Y, Dang Y. Research progress in the screening and evaluation of umami peptides. Compr Rev Food Sci Food Saf. 2022;21(2):1462–90.
27. Fan Y, Huang Y, Zhang N, Chen G, Jiang S, Zhang Y, Pang G, Wang W, Liu Y. Study on the distribution of umami receptors on the tongue and its signal coding logic based on taste bud biosensor. Biosens Bioelectron. 2022;197:113780.
28. Li M, Zhang N, Cui Z, Wang W, Wang C, Wang D, Li M, Lu W, Qing G, Liu Y. Biomimetic ion nanochannels for sensing umami substances. Biomaterials. 2022;282:121418.
29. Ahn SR, An JH, Song HS, Park JW, Lee SH, Kim JH, Jang J, Park TH. Duplex bioelectronic tongue for sensing umami and sweet tastes based on human taste receptor nanovesicles. ACS Nano. 2016;10(8):7287–96.
30. Cheng T, Li Q, Zhou Z, Wang Y, Bryant SH. Structure-based virtual screening for drug discovery: a problem-centric review. AAPS J. 2012;14(1):133–41.
31. Li X, Xie X, Wang J, Xu Y, Yi S, Zhu W, Mi H, Li T, Li J. Identification, taste characteristics and molecular docking study of novel umami peptides derived from the aqueous extract of the clam Meretrix meretrix Linnaeus. Food Chem. 2020;312:126053.
32. Zhang Y, Venkitasamy C, Pan Z, Liu W, Zhao L. Novel umami ingredients: umami peptides and their taste. J Food Sci. 2017;82(1):16–23.
33. Yamasaki Y, Maekawa K. A peptide with delicious taste. Agric Biol Chem. 2014;42(9):1761–5.
34. Wassenaar PV, Van D, Schaaper W. Taste of delicious beefy meaty peptide. Rev J Agric Food Chem. 1995;43(11):2828–32.

35. Tamura M, Nakatsuka T, Tada M, Kawasaki Y, Kikuchi E, Okai H. The relationship between taste and primary structure of "delicious peptide" (Lys-Gly-Asp-Glu-Glu-Ser-Leu-Ala) from beef soup. Agric Biol Chem. 1989;53(2):319–25.
36. Fu B, Xu X, Zhang X, Cheng S, El-Seedi HR, Du M. Identification and characterisation of taste-enhancing peptides from oysters (*Crassostrea gigas*) via the Maillard reaction. Food Chem. 2023;424:136412.
37. Spanier A, Bland J, Miller J, Glinka J, Wasz W, Duggins T. BMP: a flavor enhancing peptide found naturally in beef. Its chemical synthesis, descriptive sensory analysis, and some factors affecting its usefulness. Dev Food Sci. 1995;37.
38. Miyamura N, Iida Y, Kuroda M, Kato Y, Yamazaki J, Mizukoshi T, Miyano H. Determination and quantification of kokumi peptide, gamma-glutamyl-valyl-glycine, in brewed alcoholic beverages. J Biosci Bioeng. 2015;120(3):311–4.
39. Kuroda M, Kato Y, Yamazaki J, Kai Y, Mizukoshi T, Miyano H, Eto Y. Determination and quantification of γ-glutamyl-valyl-glycine in commercial fish sauces. J Agric Food Chem. 2012;60(29):7291–6.
40. Arai S, Yamashita M, Noguchi M, Fujimaki M. Tastes of L-glutamyl oligopeptides in relation to their chromatographic properties. Agric Biol Chem. 1973;37(1):151–6.

Chapter 10
Processing and Application of Marine Shellfish Protein

Ming Du, Shaoyun Wang, Di Wu, Shuzhen Cheng, and Huijia Yan

Abstract Marine shellfish proteins represent valuable marine bioresources whose functional and nutritional properties can be significantly enhanced through physical and biological processing. Physical methods primarily modify protein structure and particle size to enhance functionality, whereas biological approaches employ enzymatic hydrolysis to improve bioactivity and bioavailability. These processing methods provide a broader scope for the application of shellfish proteins in the food industry. Such modifications result from changes in protein particle size, solubility, emulsion stability, secondary structure, and bioactivity. Physical treatments induce phenomena including friction, collision, shear forces, turbulence, and cavitation, which alter protein particle size. Studies demonstrate that processing methods such as ultrasound, high-pressure homogenization, ball milling, and enzymatic hydrolysis modify the structural, physical, and chemical properties of food-derived proteins.

Keywords Marine shellfish protein · Modification · Enzymatic · Structure · Function · Bioactivity

Shellfish represent economically significant aquaculture products in China, with extensive cultivation history. There are nearly 20 economically significant shellfish species that have been cultured on a large scale. They contain abundant proteins, polysaccharides, unsaturated fatty acids, minerals (including iron, copper, iodine, potassium, sodium, calcium, phosphorus), vitamins, and diverse bioactive compounds, including peptides, sterols, saponins, and terpenes. They offer

M. Du (✉)
College of Food Science and Engineering, Dalian Ocean University, Dalian, China

S. Wang
Biological Science and Engineering, Fuzhou University, Fuzhou, China

D. Wu · H. Yan
Food Science and Engineering, Dalian Polytechnic University, Dalian, China

S. Cheng
School of Food Science and Technology, Dalian Polytechnic University, Dalian, China

M. Du, S. Cheng (eds.), *Bioactive Proteins and Peptides from Marine Shellfish*,
https://doi.org/10.1007/978-981-95-3937-6_10

nutritional advantages not found in terrestrial proteins, making them ideal base ingredients for food products and additives.

Current domestic research on *Chlamys farreri* (a scallop species) primarily addresses aquaculture, breeding, heavy metal detection, and condiment development from this species. However, studies on high-value product development, protein and peptide separation, purification, and characterization remain limited. Muscle proteins constitute the primary functional components in meat, governing physicochemical properties and sensory characteristics of meat products. The proteins in *Chlamys farreri* meat can generally be divided into myofibrillar proteins, sarcoplasmic proteins, and stromal proteins. Myofibrillar proteins are salt-soluble proteins, accounting for 50%–55% of the total protein content, and are divided into myosin, actin, and actomyosin. Their functional properties—water-holding capacity, emulsification, and gelation—directly influence food protein processing. Sarcoplasmic proteins (30%–35%), as water-soluble components, determine taste profiles and emulsification properties. Their myoglobin content governs meat coloration. Stromal proteins are insoluble proteins, accounting for 10%–15% of the total protein. As primary constituents of connective tissue, they contain collagen and elastin that critically influence meat tenderness and elasticity. Therefore, structural modifications in shellfish proteins directly alter their functional properties and application performance as food additives, including solubility, emulsification, foaming capacity, and gelation.

Current modification of marine shellfish proteins primarily employs traditional physical or biological methods. Compared to chemical modification, physical modification is more widely used in the food industry, which can reduce the introduction of chemical substances in the processing. Current physical techniques include ultrasound, ultrafine grinding, and high-pressure homogenization. These methods induce particle-level phenomena—friction, collision, shear forces, turbulence, and cavitation—that alter protein particle size and molecular structure. Consequently, they enhance functional properties, including surface hydrophobicity, solubility, emulsification, and gelation. Compared to physical approaches, biological modifications—microbial fermentation and enzymatic hydrolysis—offer eco-friendly and energy-efficient advantages. Simultaneously, biological processing enhances nutritional quality, functional performance, and bioavailability of proteins, garnering significant research and industrial interest.

10.1 Solubility

As large organic molecules, proteins form dispersed colloidal systems in water. Thus, conventional solubility concepts do not strictly apply. Instead, protein solubility denotes the dispersion level or amount maintained in aqueous solution. This solubility depends on conditions such as pH value, ionic strength, temperature, and solvent type. Solubility reaches its minimum at the isoelectric point (pI). At pH values above or below pI, proteins acquire net negative or positive charges, respectively, enhancing solubility. Despite this minimum solubility at pI, significant variation exists among proteins. Casein and soy protein become nearly insoluble at pI, whereas whey protein retains solubility. Proteins exhibiting strong pH-dependent solubility enable convenient extraction and separation through pH adjustment. Those with pH-stable solubility require alternative separation and purification methods. Salts differentially affect protein solubility. At 0.1–1 M concentrations, neutral salts enhance solubility *via* ionic strength effects. Conversely, concentrations exceeding 1 M reduce solubility and may induce precipitation.

Molluscan muscle proteins are categorized into three groups: (1) myofibrillar proteins (MFP, salt-soluble, 50%–55%), which include myosin, actin, and actomyosin. These proteins are characterized by water-holding capacity, fat-emulsifying properties, and gelation upon heating, playing a crucial role in meat processing (2). Sarcoplasmic proteins (water-soluble, 30%–35%), which contribute to flavor characteristics and emulsifying properties in shellfish meat and contain myoglobin, which is associated with meat color (3). Stroma proteins (insoluble, 10%–15%), including collagen and elastin, which are closely associated with meat tenderness and elasticity. Among these, myofibrillar proteins are most critical for meat product quality, as they primarily form the high-viscosity network structure within these products. Structurally, myofibrillar proteins can be further divided into three categories based on their physiological roles and organization in muscle tissue: (1) contractile proteins, primarily myosin and actin; (2) regulatory proteins, such as tropomyosin, the troponin complex, and other minor proteins; and (3) cytoskeletal (or scaffold) proteins, such as titin, nebulin, desmin, and other minor components. While some regulatory and cytoskeletal proteins influence functional properties like water retention and solubility, their primary role in improving product quality is indirect, achieved by releasing constraints on myosin and actin [1].

10.1.1 Physical Modification

Different types of products require distinct physicochemical and functional properties. In cake production, good water retention and foaming properties are essential for maintaining the structural texture. In beverage production, the solubility and emulsifying capacity of proteins are leveraged to create uniform and stable nutritional health drinks. In meat product manufacturing, the gelling ability and water-holding capacity of proteins are crucial. Protein modification involves using biochemical factors (chemical reagents, enzymatic preparations, etc.) or physical factors (heating, mechanic, etc.) to induce changes in amino acid residues and peptide chains, resulting in changes to the spatial structure and physicochemical properties of protein macromolecules, ultimately yielding improved functional and nutritional characteristics. Protein modification methods fall into three categories: physical modification, chemical modification, and enzymatic modification. Compared with other modification methods, physical modification offers advantages such as low cost, safety, and minimal impact on nutritional quality. Physical modification primarily employs ultra-fine grinding, ultrasonic treatment, homogenization, extrusion, stirring, heating, microwave treatment, and other physical methods to alter the structure, physicochemical properties, and functional properties of proteins.

The functional properties of proteins refer to the physical and chemical properties that affect their performance during production, processing, and storage; they fall into the following three types: (1) hydration properties, including solubility, water-holding capacity, oil-holding capacity, wettability, swelling capacity, adhesion, and viscosity, depend on the interaction between protein molecules and water (2). Protein aggregation properties, such as gelation and film-forming properties, involve interactions between proteins (3). Interfacial properties are primarily associated with surface tension (as influenced by proteins), emulsifying capacity, and foaming ability. The solubility of proteins is primarily linked to the hydrophobicity of protein surfaces, charge density, and the degree of protein denaturation, while gelation and emulsifying properties are primarily linked to protein solubility, molecular weight distribution, the ratio of hydrophilic and hydrophobic groups, and the content of disulfide bonds. Currently, physical processing such as ultrasonic treatment, ultra-fine grinding, and high-pressure homogenization is used for pretreatment of proteins, inducing complex friction, collision, shearing, vortices, and cavitation of protein particles, thereby altering the size and molecular structure of protein particles, subsequently improving proteins' molecular surface hydrophobicity, solubility, emulsifying properties, and gelation properties—a development that has garnered widespread attention from academia and industry.

Myosin, the primary protein in marine shellfish, is a fibrous high-molecular-weight protein with a molecular weight of approximately 500 kDa. It is the most abundant protein in myofibrils, accounting for approximately 43% of myofibrillar proteins. It consists of two myosin heavy chains (MHC) and four myosin light chains (MLC). A segment of the two heavy chains intertwines to form an α-helical rod domain, while the remaining segments, together with the four light chains, form two globular head domains. This configuration gives the molecule an overall shape commonly described as resembling a bean sprout (Fig. 10.1). The myosin molecule contains two hinge regions that enable it to bind flexibly with actin during muscle

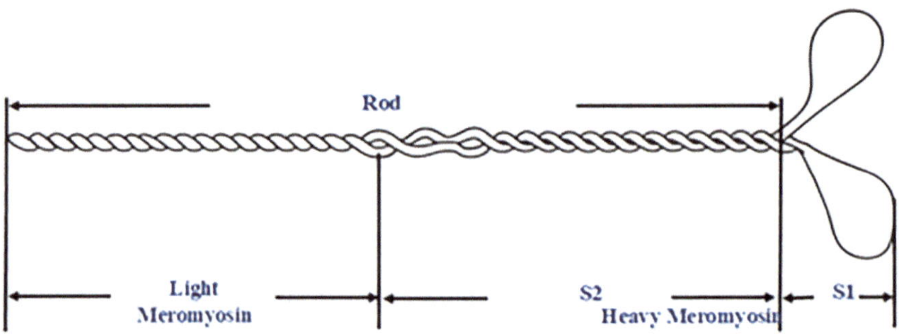

Fig. 10.1 Schematic diagram of myosin molecules in muscle. Heavy meromyosin (HMM)/light meromyosin (LMM) and S1 (subfragment 1)/Rod, where HMM can be further hydrolyzed into S1 and S2 under the action of papain

contraction. When acted upon by restrictive enzymes, the myosin molecule can be hydrolyzed at the hinge regions into several fragments: heavy meromyosin (HMM), light meromyosin (LMM), S1 (subfragment 1), and Rod. HMM can be further hydrolyzed into S1 and S2 by papain. S1 exhibits ATPase activity, is responsible for binding to actin, and the rod segment is a component of the thick filament [2, 3].

Myosin molecules consist of approximately 4500 amino acids. They exhibit a very low content of helix-breaking residues, such as proline and glycine, which disrupt α-helical structures. The molecule contains abundant charged amino acid residues: positively charged residues like arginine and lysine and negatively charged residues like aspartic acid and glutamic acid. The distribution of these residues differs significantly between domains. The Rod domain possesses a higher concentration of charged residues compared to the S1 head domain, which is relatively richer in hydrophobic amino acids. Specifically, lysine and glutamine content in the Rod is 6.6% and 4.7%, respectively—considerably higher than in S1 (4.0% and 1.8%). Myosin contains 40 cysteine residues. The sulfhydryl groups (thiol groups) of these cysteines are highly susceptible to oxidation by reactive oxygen species. This oxidation readily forms disulfide bonds, leading to protein aggregation and a consequent decrease in solubility [4].

Protein solubility, one of the most critical hydration properties, directly influences other functional properties, including emulsifying capacity and gelling ability. During the production of commercial protein powders, solubility is frequently influenced by temperature, pH, and processing techniques. Protein gelation refers to the process by which protein molecules aggregate to a critical extent and form an ordered protein network. This network reflects the electrostatic balance between attractive and repulsive forces among amino acid side chains, embodying interactions either between proteins themselves or between proteins and their solvent environment. Globular proteins (e.g., soy protein) and helical-structured proteins (e.g., myofibrillar proteins) are prime examples of proteins with excellent gelling properties. Soy proteins deform when heated, with their globular molecules unfolding into linear structures, whereas myofibrillar proteins undergo helix-destabilization during processing. This leads to amino acid residue interactions *via* heat induction or other processing techniques. Hydrophobic functional groups previously buried internally become exposed. Following processing, system disorderliness increases, molecular thermal motion intensifies, and the frequency of molecular collisions rises [5].

Chemical modification is effective, but its application is limited. This is due to three key factors: the degradation of protein nutritional value, the potential formation of harmful or toxic by-products, and concerns about reagent toxicity and residues. Enzymatic hydrolysis modification, despite its mild reaction conditions and fewer harmful by-products, is less effective at low hydrolysis degrees. Furthermore, the bitter peptides generated at high hydrolysis degrees reduce protein product palatability. Physical modification is often favored because it produces no toxic side effects, minimally impacts protein nutrition, and is low-cost. However, its overall effectiveness requires further investigation. This approach primarily employs physical techniques such as ultra-micronization, ultrasonication, homogenization, extrusion, stirring, heating, microwave treatment, and others to alter protein structure,

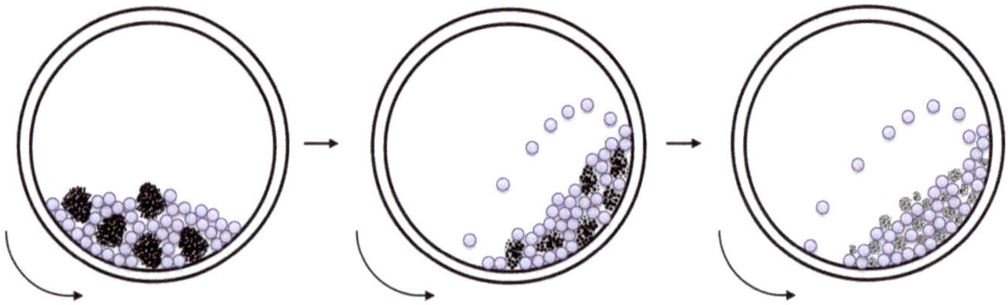

Fig. 10.2 Schematic diagram of the principle of ball mill treatment [7]

physicochemical characteristics, and functional properties. It significantly influences the molecular aggregation behavior of most proteins.

10.1.1.1 Ball Milling Treatment

Ball milling can reduce protein particle size to an average diameter of 1 nm to 100 μm. Particles reduced below 10 μm exhibit significantly increased specific surface area, porosity, and surface energy. Particle size significantly influences the physical properties, functional characteristics, and certain chemical properties of food biomaterials. Brown and Heron first demonstrated that starch particles can be physically crushed using mechanical equipment such as ball mills. This process generates mechanical forces and chemical effects *via* collision, friction, and shear. The mechanochemical effects generated by ball milling treatment may alter the conformational structure of proteins (Fig. 10.2). Wu observed that scallop protein powder particle size decreased significantly after 8–10 min of ball milling, while particle surfaces became smoother (Fig. 10.3) [3]. Following milling, additional hydrophobic groups within the protein molecules are exposed. Protein molecules accumulate at the oil–water interface, orienting their hydrophobic moieties toward the nonpolar phase and hydrophilic moieties toward the polar phase. Wang treated oyster protein powder with ultrafine grinding (ball milling) for 0, 2, 4, 6, 8, and 10 min, and scanning electron microscopy observed that the protein particles significantly decreased in size after treatment [6].

10.1.1.2 Ultrasound

Ultrasound, defined as sound waves exceeding 20 kHz (beyond human hearing), exhibits both wave propagation and energy transfer characteristics. It can be categorized into low-frequency (20–100 kHz) and high-frequency (100–1000 kHz) ultrasound. Beyond industrial applications like welding (15–40 kHz) and cleaning (20–40 kHz), ultrasound serves as a key physical processing technique (20–100 kHz) for characterizing food proteins. Appropriate modification treatments can improve the structural and functional properties of shellfish proteins, thereby enhancing the

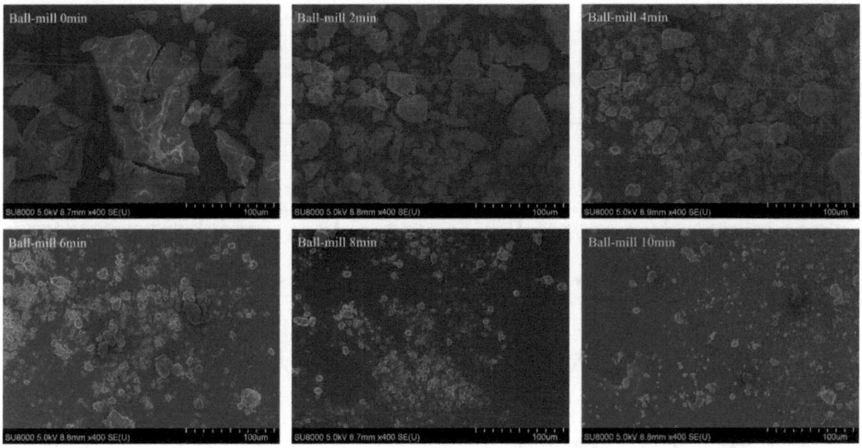

Fig. 10.3 Effects of ball milling time (0, 2, 4, 6, 8, and 10 min) on the microstructure of *Chlamys farreri* protein [4]

utilization value of this high-quality marine resource. Myofibrillar proteins, constituting 50%–55% of shellfish muscle protein, represent a primary research focus in food protein processing. Ultrasound modifies proteins primarily through cavitation, which generates intense physical forces—including shear, shock waves, and turbulence—that alter protein functional properties. During operation, an ultrasonic transducer generates intense localized pressure around the probe tip. This pressure rapidly collapses cavitation bubbles, releasing energy as heat, microjets, and shock waves that disrupt surrounding material and facilitate gas release (Fig. 10.4) [7].

During food processing, ultrasound induces water vapor decomposition, generating hydroxyl radicals (·OH) and hydrogen atoms (Ḥ). These reactive species initiate redox reactions that degrade proteins and inactivate enzymes, ultimately enhancing protein functionality [8]. Ultrasound technology, as a nonthermal processing method in the food industry, has garnered widespread attention for its ability to develop mild processes that yield higher quality and safer food products. Soria demonstrated that 200 kHz ultrasound treatment enhances solubility, flowability, and stability in myofibrillar protein suspensions [8, 9]. Intense shear, impact forces, and cavitation disrupt myofibrillar proteins, causing dissociation into fibers, oligomers, and myosin monomers. This structural disassembly enhances solubility, particularly for hydrophobic proteins [10].

Pulsed ultrasound pretreatment (20 kHz; 20%–40% amplitude) increases surface hydrophobicity in cuttlefish (*Dosidicus gigas*) proteins, enhancing their adsorption capacity at oil–water interfaces This increased hydrophobicity raised the emulsifying activity index from 123.67 ± 5.52 m^2/g to 217.70 ± 3.80 m^2/g, improving both emulsifying activity and stability [11]. Jambrak found that ultrasound treatment (20 kHz) plays a significant role in the functional properties of whey proteins such as solubility and foaming ability. Treatments at 40 kHz produced weaker effects than 20 kHz, while 500 kHz ultrasound showed negligible impact. The results

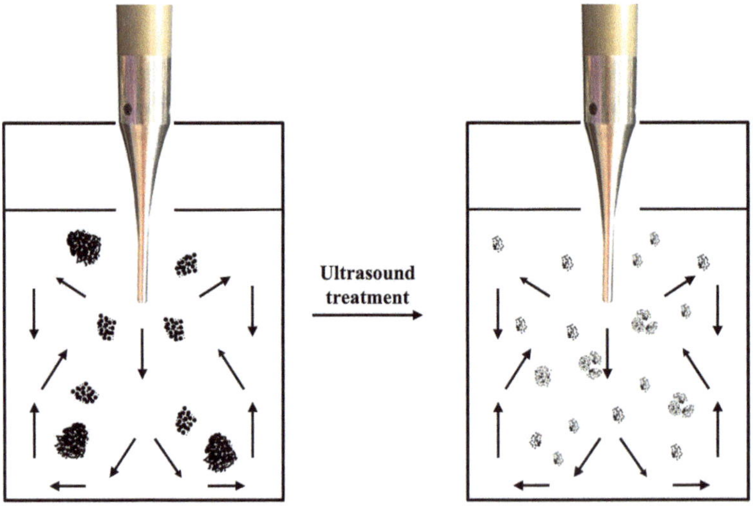

Fig. 10.4 Schematic diagram of the principle of ultrasound treatment. Sonication similarly reduced the size of protein aggregates due to disruption of noncovalent interactions similarly displayed growth of particle size attributed to increases in temperature, resulting in protein denaturation and aggregation [7]

indicate that the appropriate use of ultrasound power and time can positively affect the product. Additionally, it was found that whey proteins treated with 20 and 40 kHz ultrasound experienced a significant reduction in particle size and molecular weight [12]. Chen observed that increasing ultrasound duration (10–30 min) and power (100–300 W) elevated pH in myofibrillar proteins, enhancing water-holding capacity and gel strength. Maximum improvement occurred at 300 W and 30 min. At the same time, emulsifying properties were improved due to the significant reduction in particle size. Wu reported significantly improved dispersibility and increased nitrogen solubility index in scallop proteins after 600–950 W ultrasound treatment (Fig. 10.5) [10].

10.1.1.3 High-Pressure Homogenization

High-pressure homogenization (HPH) is a continuous nonthermal processing technology suitable for fluid materials. During HPH, proteins experience intense shear, turbulence, cavitation, and thermal effects within the homogenizing valve, disrupting noncovalent bonds. This leads to structural rearrangement of the proteins, driven by intramolecular and intermolecular forces, thereby altering the physicochemical properties and functional characteristics of the proteins. HPH is favored for its ease of operation, scalability, reproducibility, and high throughput, making it one of the most suitable technologies for industrial applications. Optimized HPH treatment enhances protein structure and functionality, with mussel proteins showing particular promise for nutritious food development. The HPH process involves subjecting

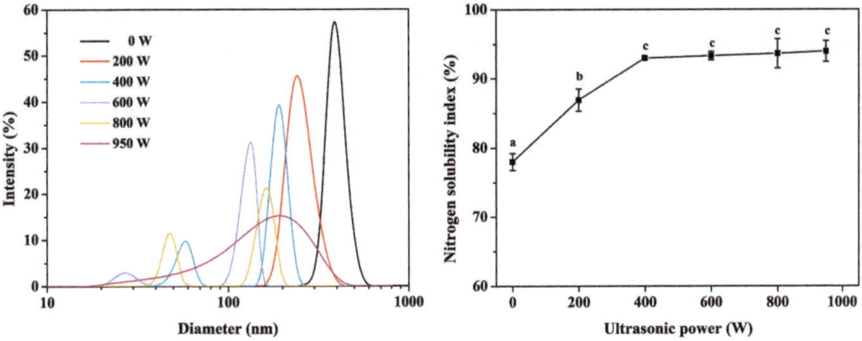

Fig. 10.5 Effects of ultrasound treatments (0, 200, 400, 600, 800, and 950 W) on the particle size distribution (**a**) and nitrogen solubility index (**b**) of *Chlamys farreri* protein [10]

fluid materials to high pressure, which then pass through an adjustable narrow gap (≤2 μm), causing a pressure drop to atmospheric pressure. The pressure differential accelerates fluid velocity, generating homogenizing and thermal effects that alter product physicochemical properties.

HPH is a continuous, nonthermal processing technology suitable for fluid foods. During HPH, proteins undergo significant changes due to deformation caused by intense pressure. This affects molecular bonds, leading to their breakage and reorganization, thereby altering protein functionality. The physical properties of the homogenized material are altered depending on the material's characteristics, applied pressure level, and treatment duration. Based on pressure intensity, homogenization is categorized into two types: HPH with pressures up to 300 MPa and ultra-high-pressure homogenization (UHPH) operating between 350 and 400 MPa. HPH enables continuous production, scalable from laboratory bench-scale units to industrial-scale systems exceeding 10,000 L/h.

Currently, industrial, pilot, or laboratory-scale high-pressure homogenizers typically consist of a high-pressure pump (piston type) and an interruption valve or nozzle made of wear-resistant ceramics or hard gemstones. During HPH, piston pumps propel fluid samples through a narrow orifice. At the valve gap exit, the fluid undergoes rapid acceleration, generating turbulence, cavitation, and impact forces. The physical stresses induced by HPH can lead to significant structural changes in proteins, improving their performance as ingredients (e.g., increasing solubility, water retention, and emulsifying capacity).

HPH, operating parameters such as homogenization pressure, homogenization temperature, number of homogenization cycles or passes, valve design, and homogenization flow rate are important factors that affect the performance of homogenization. During processing, temperature rises linearly with pressure due to adiabatic heating at the valve. This thermal effect results from pressure application, turbulence, shear forces, and cavitation during pressure release downstream. Depending on fluid compressibility, this increase approximates 16–20 °C per 100 MPa. Although materials with small particle size do not undergo thermal degradation within the valve due to the short residence time, the frictional heat generated in the homogenizer can significantly affect the physicochemical properties of food proteins, especially during multiple or continuous HPH treatment processes. To minimize heating deterioration, HPH processes typically use low inlet temperatures and rapid cooling at the fluid outlet. Jet valves, based on the impact of two turbulent flows, have the advantage of having no moving parts, which simplifies operation. One renowned HPH equipment that uses this type of valve is the microfluidic system established by Microfluidics.

As shown in Fig. 10.6, the radial expansion valve features an axial valve face and movable valve seat that regulates homogenization pressure by adjusting slit width and upstream flow rate. The GEA Niro Soavi homogenizer exemplifies equipment utilizing radial diffusion valves. Pilot systems from Microfluidics (US) and GEA Niro Soavi (Italy) achieve homogenization pressures up to 200 MPa with average flow rates of 160 L/h. HPH modifies food proteins through top-down (particle size reduction) or bottom-up (particle reorganization) processes, conferring novel structures and physicochemical properties. This creates opportunities for tailored protein functionality enhancement in customized products [7].

High-pressure homogenization represents an extensively studied emulsification technique and critical unit operation for producing uniformly dispersed emulsions. Its generated mechanical forces both fragment oil droplets into uniform dispersions and induce protein conformational changes. These altered proteins adsorb onto newly formed oil droplet surfaces, enhancing emulsion stability. HPH unfolds myofibrillar protein helical structures and promotes myosin oligomerization *via* disulfide bonding. This conformational shift inhibits thin filament formation, improving myofibrillar protein solubility. HPH can be used to improve the functional properties of mussel isolate proteins, broadening their application in mussel isolate protein products. Wu recovered mussel isolate proteins using isoelectric precipitation and

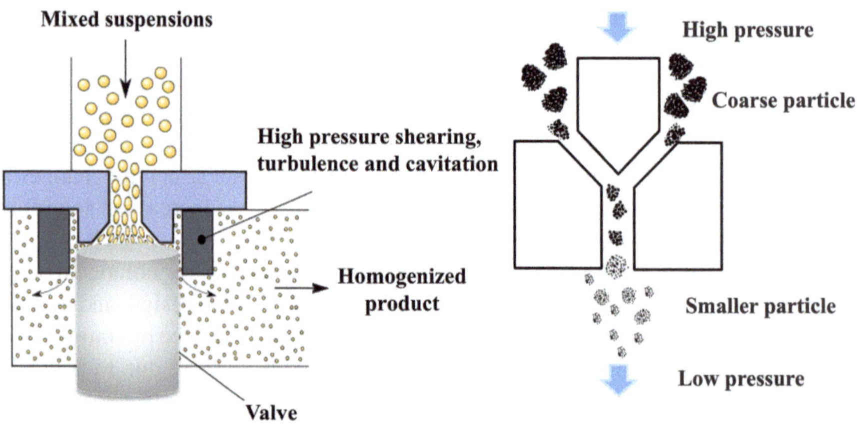

Fig. 10.6 High-pressure homogenization. Mixed suspensions were loaded into the channel of high-pressure homogenization, which may reduce the size and alter the morphology of particles through a combination of high-pressure shearing, turbulence, and cavitation effects, resulting in different particle shapes [7]

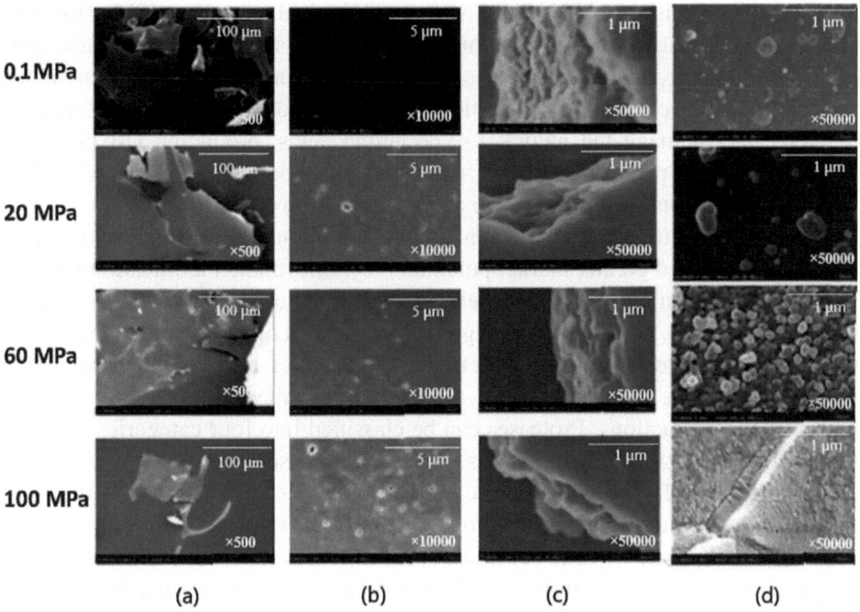

Fig. 10.7 High-pressure homogenization on the surface properties of oyster protein powder [16]

treated the protein solution under pressures of 20, 40, 60, 80, and 100 MPa in a high-pressure homogenizer (GEA Niro Soavi, Panda Plus 2000). The content of free sulfhydryl groups slightly increased within the pressure range of 0–40 MPa but showed a decreasing trend at higher HPH pressures [14]. As the pressure increases from 20 to 100 MPa, surface hydrophobicity tends to increase due to the stretching and unfolding of protein molecules. The absolute zeta potential of proteins increases at pressures between 20–60 MPa and decreases at 80–100 MPa, with a broader particle size distribution observed, attributed to the formation of aggregates (Fig. 10.7) [16].

10.1.2 Chemical and Biological Modification

Protein chemical modification fundamentally involves functionalizing main-chain or side-chain groups to alter protein spatial configurations and physicochemical properties. Common methods include glycosylation, oxidation, phosphorylation, and covalent cross-linking. By modifying functional groups such as amino, hydroxyl, carboxyl, or thiol groups in the peptide chain, the purpose of protein modification is achieved [17]. Protein glycosylation is the process where sugars, under the influence of enzymes, covalently bond with protein residues to form glycosidic bonds. The highly hydrophilic sugar groups affect the physicochemical and functional properties of proteins. Glycosylation of proteins also has important biological functions; it not only influences the structure and stability of proteins but also plays an indispensable role in various biological processes [18]. However, chemical modification poses limitations: it may compromise nutritional value, generate harmful byproducts, and leave toxic reagent residues. There have been numerous reports on the chemical modification of proteins to date. Chemical modification methods may damage the natural L-type amino acids, producing D-type amino acids and harmful proline derivatives. Moreover, the modification involves covalent bonding interactions, requiring rather stringent reaction conditions.

Protein bioreactors require mild enzymatic conditions (pH 6.0–8.0, temperature 40–60 °C) and hold greater market potential [19]. Enzymatic modification substantially alters protein structures, with effects dependent on substrate characteristics, enzyme specificity, and hydrolysis degree. Strict control of hydrolysis extent is critical: excessive cleavage impairs functionality, generates bitter peptides, increases ionic components, and enhances hydrophobicity—collectively altering protein–environment interactions. Proteases can be classified into four categories based on their active centers: serine proteases, cysteine proteases, aspartic proteases, and metalloproteases. In mammals, serine proteases play a significant role, with activation achieved through changes in a group of amino acid residues in the active center, one of which is always serine. Pepsin and pancreatic enzymes such as chymotrypsin and trypsin are all serine proteases. Pepsin tends to cleave peptide bonds at the amino or carboxy termini that are aromatic amino acids or leucine; it does not effectively cleave if the peptide starts from the C-terminus with the third amino acid being a basic amino acid or if the N-terminus is arginine. The main components of pancreatic enzymes are chymotrypsin, which is a peptide chain endoenzyme, and trypsin, which is a hydrolase enzyme. Chymotrypsin primarily cleaves hydrophobic amino acid carboxy termini, while trypsin promotes peptide chain splitting at the carboxy groups of arginine or lysine. Evidence confirms serine proteases enhance protein solubility, emulsification, and gelation properties [20].

Research indicates that proteolytic enzymes catalyze complexation reactions in protein–peptide mixtures, enhancing bioactive and nutritional properties [21, 22]. Controlled enzymatic hydrolysis induces conformational changes in aquatic proteins: globular structures unfold, exposing buried hydrophobic groups. This elevated surface hydrophobicity promotes protein aggregation and subsequent gelation—a phenomenon specific to enzyme–substrate–hydrolysis degree combinations. Enzyme selection critically determines hydrolysate characteristics, as modifications directly depend on protease specificity. Strict hydrolysis control remains essential, since excessive cleavage impairs functionality and generates bitter peptides. Enzymatic treatment reduces molecular weight, increases ionizable groups, enhances hydrophobicity, and alters protein–environment interactions. Male *Patinopecten yessoensis* protein hydrolysates have good solubility and potential application prospects in formulated food systems [23]. Mannheim demonstrated this by hydrolyzing proteins at 50 °C (pH 8–9) for 0–4 h with 0–1.75 mg/mL protease, achieving 90%–92% solubility, water-holding capacity increases from 0.2 to 3.75 g/g, and significantly enhanced foaming properties [24].

Yuan demonstrated that high-pressure homogenization (30 MPa) combined with pepsin hydrolysis (pH 2.0, 37 °C, 30 min) maximized protein solubility at pH 2–4 while increasing foaming capacity by 65% [25]. Separately, Avano treated shellfish proteins with alkaline protease (substrate-to-enzyme ratio 1:100, pH 8.5, 60 °C, 30 min), elevating solubility from 8.25% to 22.14% [26]. Therefore, enzyme-modified bioreactors are widely applied in the industrial processing of proteins. This targeted process cleaves peptide bonds to alter amino acid sequences and restructure proteins. A significant advantage of enzymatic hydrolysis is that it preserves the original chemical components extracted from food, which positively affects the nutritional value and functional properties of proteins in food processing. Compared to native proteins, hydrolysates exhibit superior digestibility, gastrointestinal absorption, and organoleptic properties.

10.1.3 Heat

Heat treatment is a common processing technique in the food industry, including methods such as cooking, thermal sterilization, and spray drying, which are widely applied in industrial production. Heat treatment is also one of the commonly used technical means to improve the functional properties of proteins [14]. Heat treatment above the denaturation temperature often leads to protein unfolding, exposing some groups buried within the protein molecules, which subsequently leads to protein aggregation and the formation of protein gels.

In recent years, the changes in the physicochemical properties of proteins and their thermal aggregation behavior during heat treatment have received widespread attention. Guo observed that thermal treatment reduced solubility of oyster protein isolates, reaching minimum levels at 60 °C before increasing at 100 °C—suggesting possible thermal degradation effects (Fig. 10.8). Reactive oxygen can directly induce the oxidation of the protein main chain and side chains, leading to the breakage of the protein main chain and side-chain β-scission. The decrease in protein solubility after heat treatment may affect the subsequent utilization of oyster salt-soluble proteins [15]. Zhang observed with confocal microscopy that differently sized native oyster water-soluble proteins were dispersed in the solution in a flaky structure with very short inter-particle distances. Due to their low electronegativity, oyster water-soluble proteins come close to each other in the solution to form protein clusters [12, 27]. After heating at 45 °C, oyster water-soluble proteins exhibit partial aggregation, whereas untreated oyster water-soluble proteins are more uniformly distributed. Heat treatment exposes hydrophobic residues within the oyster proteins, leading to protein denaturation and the formation of polymers [27]. Further heat treatment results in the formation of extensive disulfide bonds within the oyster proteins, making the flaky oyster water-soluble protein structure more compact. Consequently, no larger aggregation is observed at higher temperatures [26] (Table 10.1).

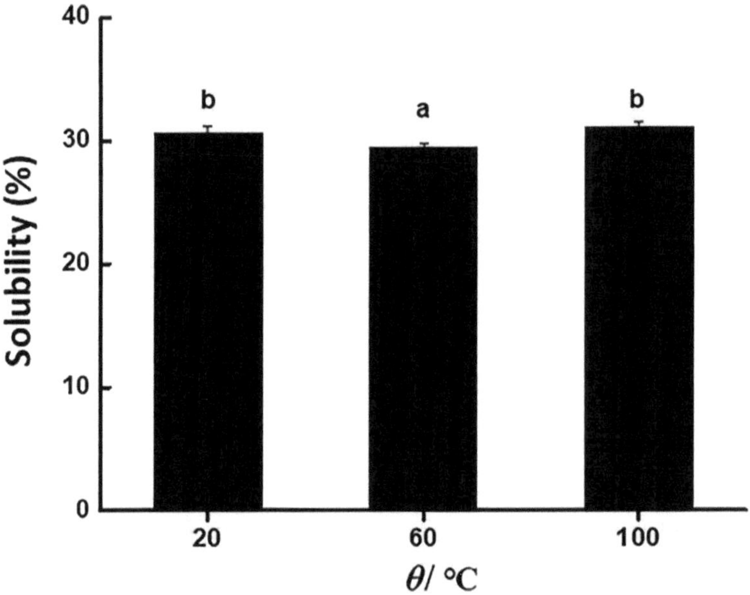

Fig. 10.8 Effects of heat treatment on the solubility of oyster protein at different temperatures (20, 60, 100 °C)

10.2 Water-Holding Capacity and Oil-Holding Capacity

Proteins are amphiphilic macromolecules composed of α-amino acids connected *via* peptide bonds. Their water or oil retention capacity reflects the ability to absorb and retain these solvents within their structural matrix. Protein-bound water exhibits distinct physicochemical properties compared to bulk water due to solvent–biomolecule interactions. This binding behavior is primarily governed by the polarity and density of hydrophilic groups within the protein. Key factors influencing protein-water binding include amino acid composition, conformational state, surface characteristics, pH, temperature, and ionic environment.

10.2.1 Physical Modification

Moderate ultrasonication (<600 W) yields gels with dense, uniform cavities that firmly immobilize water molecules within the network, resisting centrifugal expulsion. However, exceeding 600 W creates larger, unstable cavities where water is loosely trapped, facilitating release during centrifugation and reducing water-holding capacity. Therefore, both the protein charge and the microstructure of myofibrillar protein gels play significant roles in the water retention process, which is consistent with the previously proposed hypothesis [34, 35]. Wu subjected scallop

Table 10.1 Effects of physical treatment on shellfish proteins

No.	Protein	Characterization	Parameters	References
1	Mussel (*Mytilus edulis*) protein hydrolysis	The controlled enzymatic hydrolysis of mussel protein with trypsin, followed by the enzyme solution being mixed with multiple ratios of additives such as complex polysaccharides, carrageenan, sodium carboxymethyl cellulose, and xanthan gum, has improved the solubility of mussel protein	Mussel protein (50 g) was put in 150 mL of distilled water (1:3 w/v) and digest it with trypsin (5000 U/g) at pH 8.5 and 45 °C for 2 h. Adjust and maintain a constant pH using 1 M hydrochloric acid and 0.5 M sodium hydroxide	[29]
2	Scallops (*Chlamys farreri*) protein	Subject scallop protein powder to ball milling for 0, 2, 4, 6, 8, and 10 min, and then perform in vitro simulated digestion of the samples after different ball milling durations. The nitrogen solubility index increased from 42.01 ± 0.31% in the untreated sample to 58.78 ± 3.37%	Protein was put into a ball mill (MM400, Retsch Technology, Haan, Germany) at 20 Hz with a P8 setting for 0, 2, 4, 6, 8, and 10 min. After ball milling, treat the samples with pepsin at pH 2.0 at an enzyme-to-substrate ratio of 3:100 for 1 h. After pepsin digested, proceed with trypsin digestion at pH 7.0 at an E/S of 3:100 for 4 h. following the inactivation of trypsin, centrifuge the samples at 10,000× *g* for 20 min	[30]
3	Oyster (*Crassostrea gigas*) protein	Subject oyster protein powder to ultra-micro pulverization (ball milling) for 0, 2, 4, 6, 8, and 10 min, and then perform in vitro simulated digestion of the samples after different ball milling durations. SEM observations show that the protein particles are significantly reduced in size after treatment	Ball-mill (MM400, Retsch Technology, Haan, Germany), 20 Hz, P8, (0, 4, 8, 12, 16, 20 min)	[28]
4	Scallops (*Chlamys farreri*) protein hydrolysis	Subject the scallop protein powder to ultra-micro pulverization (ball milling) for 10 min, and then perform in vitro simulated digestion and enzymatic hydrolysis	Protein powder was placed into a ball mill (MM400, Retsch Technology, Haan, Germany) and perform ball milling at 20 Hz with a P8 setting for 10 min. After that, subject the treated samples to pepsin digestion at pH 2.0 with an enzyme-to-substrate ratio of 3:100 for 1 h. After inactivating the pepsin, proceed with trypsin digestion at pH 7.0 with an enzyme-to-substrate ratio of 3:100 for 4 h. following the inactivation of trypsin, centrifuge the samples at 10,000× *g* for 20 min	[30]

(continued)

Table 10.1 (continued)

No.	Protein	Characterization	Parameters	References
5	Scallops (*Chlamys farreri*) protein	Subject scallop protein powder to ultrasonic treatment at 0, 200, 400, 600, 800, and 950 W. After treatment at 950 W, the protein solubility increased from the original untreated level of 80.98 ± 0.82% to 93.96 ± 0.52%	An ultrasonic disruptor (Ningbo Scientz Biotechnology Co., China) was used to treat 100 mL of scallop protein solution (0.5%, w/v) with a probe diameter of 0.636 cm at ultrasonic powers of 0, 200, 400, 600, 800, and 950 W (ultrasound for 2 s, pause for 2 s), with corresponding ultrasonic intensities of 0, 707.71, 1415.43, 2123.14, 2830.86 and 3361.64 W cm^{-2}	[4]
6	Mussel (*Mytilus edulis*) protein	After treating mussel myofibrillar protein at 80 MPa, the zeta potential, emulsifying activity index, emulsion stability index, foaming ability, and foaming stability increased by 23.64 mV, 14.99 m^2/g, 4.3 min, 17.3%, and 29.7%, respectively; after treating mussel myofibrillar protein at 100 MPa, the protein solubility increased by 7.4%	HPH (GEA Niro Soavi model Panda Plus 2000, Parma, Italy) 0, 20, 40, 60, 80, and 100 MPa for 3 times	[29]
7	Oysters (*Magallana gigas*) protein	High-pressure homogenization (HPH) pretreatment enhanced the trypsin hydrolysis degree of oyster protein, resulting in a decrease in protein particle size and an increase in solubility	Utilize a high-pressure homogenizer (GEA Niro Soavi model Panda Plus 2000, Parma, Italy) to cyclically treat oyster protein solutions (10–50 mg/mL, pH 7.0) at pressures ranging from 0 to 100 MPa for two cycles	[31]
8	Oysters (*Magallana gigas*) protein	After high-pressure homogenization treatment of the oyster protein solution, the protein solubility increased from the original untreated level of 20.24%–57.99%	Utilize a high-pressure homogenizer (GEA Niro Soavi model Panda Plus 2000, Parma, Italy) to treat oyster protein solutions at pressures of 0, 20, 40, 60, 80, and 100 MPa in three cycles	[32]
9	Mussel (*Mytilus edulis*) protein	As the power increases, the solubility gradually increases, but there is no significant difference in solubility between 30 and 60 min at the same power level	Use an ultrasonic disruptor (Ningbo Scientz Biotechnology Co., China) to treat 100 mL of scallop protein solution (0.5%, w/v) with a probe diameter of 0.636 cm at ultrasonic powers of 200, 400, and 600 W (ultrasound for 2 s, pause for 2 s), with treatment times of 18 and 36 min	[6]

10	Oysters (*Magallana gigas*) protein	Acid treatment leads to the dissociation and unfolding of oyster proteins, and controlled enzymatic hydrolysis technology, high-pressure homogenization (HPH), and their combined treatments significantly improve the functional properties of oyster proteins, increasing their solubility. The emulsifying and foaming properties of proteins treated with acid or controlled enzymatic hydrolysis technology are also significantly improved	Minced oyster meat is dispersed in deionized water (1:3, w/v), and the pH is adjusted to 10.0 with 1 M NaOH. Stir at 25°C for 2 h, then centrifuge at 10,000× *g* for 15 min. The supernatant is divided into two parts. One part is adjusted to pH 5.0 with 1 M HCl, maintained for 1 h, and then centrifuged at 10,000× *g* for 10 min. The precipitate is redispersed in deionized water, neutralized to pH 7.0 with 1 M NaOH, and then freeze-dried. The other part of the supernatant is adjusted to pH 2.0 with 1 M HCl and stirred at 25 °C for 1 h. Component 1: Acid-treated oyster protein solution after treatment with a solution at pH 2.0; component 2: HPH treatment: pH 2.0, 60 MPa for three cycles; component 3: acid treatment combined with limited proteolysis: the oyster protein solution at pH 2.0 is hydrolyzed with pepsin at 37 °C for 15 min; component 4: Acid combined with limited proteolysis and HPH treatment: after AT-LP treatment, it is processed with HPH at 60 MPa for three cycles	[31]
11	False abalone (*Volutharpa ampullacea perryi*)	Enzymatic hydrolysis of abalone was carried out using pepsin, alkaline protease, neutral protease, and flavor enzyme. Compared to trypsin, pepsin showed the highest degree of hydrolysis and the strongest ability to scavenge ABTS+ free radicals. Response surface methodology was used to study the pepsin hydrolysis reaction, indicating that there is an interdependent relationship among hydrolysis temperature, time, and pH. The response surface experiment was optimized at 51.8 °C, 4.1 h, and pH 7.7	According to the GB/T5009.3-2016 and GB/T5009.5-2016 standards, the moisture content of the pseudo-abalone samples was determined to be 77.53 ± 2.13%, and the protein content was 18.24 ± 1.03%. Enzymatic hydrolysis of abalone meat was carried out using five types of proteases: pepsin (400 U/mg protein), alkaline protease (200 U/mg protein), trypsin (2500 U/mg protein), neutral protease (600 U/mg protein), and flavor enzyme (300 U/mg protein). The abalone samples were mixed at a ratio of 3% (w/v) in buffer solutions with pH levels of 2.0, 7.0, 8.0, and 10.0. Each of the five proteases was added at a ratio of 7% (w/v)	[31]

(continued)

Table 10.1 (continued)

No.	Protein	Characterization	Parameters	References
12	Mussel (*Mytilus edulis*) protein	Separate the different tissues and organs of mussels into the following parts: foot, byssus, adductor muscle, mantle, gills, retractor muscle, and visceral mass. Analyze the basic composition of proteins and other indicators for each part. After identification by QTOF-MS/MS, molecular simulation is conducted using Discovery Studio, and the enzymatic hydrolysis products are found to have potential anticoagulant activity	Utilize trypsin (25,000 U/mg protein) to enzymatically hydrolyze various tissues and organs of mussels, including the foot, byssus, adductor muscle, mantle, gills, retractor muscle, and visceral mass, at 45 °C. The tissues are mixed at a ratio of 2% (w/v) in a buffer solution with a pH of 8.5 for the enzymatic hydrolysis process	[32]
13	Mussel (*Mytilus edulis*) protein	The hydrolysis degree of different protein fractions was determined. The salt-soluble protein fraction showed a higher degree of hydrolysis (DH) compared to the other two protein fractions, and enzymatic hydrolysis increased the solubility of both salt-soluble and water-soluble proteins	Utilize trypsin (5000 U/mg protein) at 45 °C for the enzymatic hydrolysis of mussel salt-soluble proteins and water-soluble proteins. The mussel protein samples are mixed at a ratio of 2% (w/v) in a buffer solution with a pH of 8.5 for enzymatic hydrolysis, and the degree of hydrolysis is measured over a period of 3 h	[33]

protein powder to ultra-micro pulverization (ball milling) for 0, 2, 4, 6, 8, and 10 min, and then performed in vitro simulated digestion of the samples after different ball milling durations. This treatment resulted in an increase in the nitrogen solubility index of the protein solution after simulated digestion from 42.01 ± 0.31% in the untreated samples to 58.78 ± 3.37% [4].

10.2.2 Biotechnological Modification

Seafood protein hydrolysates demonstrate excellent water- and oil-holding capacities, enhancing cooking yields when incorporated into meat emulsions. Jin et al. investigated the hydrolysate of male scallop gonads with a material-to-liquid ratio of 1:20, where the mixture was heated to 95 °C for 10 min to remove denatured proteins. After neutral protease hydrolysis and freeze-drying, they evaluated the water-binding and oil-binding capabilities of the hydrolysate from male scallop gonads as a functional ingredient in meat products [36]. The water-holding capacity of scallop gonads significantly increased after enzymatic hydrolysis. This enhancement correlates with exposed polar groups (–COOH, $-NH_2$) generated during hydrolysis. Due to the increased solubility of scallop gonad hydrolysates, extensive hydrolysis can reduce their water-holding and oil-binding capacities. Hydrolysates of scallop gonads with a lower degree of hydrolysis may be effective components in certain foods that are important for water and oil binding [37]. Mao conducted controlled enzymatic hydrolysis of mussel proteins using trypsin, and the hydrolysate was mixed with additives such as complex polysaccharides, carrageenan, sodium carboxymethyl cellulose, and xanthan gum in multiple ratios, which improved the stability of mussel protein solutions [36, 37].

10.3 Emulsifying Properties

Emulsification involves stabilizing immiscible liquids (e.g., oil–water) at their interface. Without surfactants, these liquids separate by density, forming distinct layers [29]. When an appropriate surfactant is added and the mixture is vigorously stirred, the oil is dispersed in water to form an emulsion, a process known as emulsification. The emulsifying properties of proteins are an important functional characteristic, including emulsifying activity and emulsion stability. Emulsion stability refers to the ability of an emulsion to maintain a distinctly stable state without exhibiting signs of phase separation or instability. Factors that typically affect emulsion stability include emulsifying equipment, emulsifying temperature, emulsifying time, and stirring speed. Emulsion stability relies on electrostatic repulsion, which is due to the adsorption of emulsifiers around emulsion particles, imparting a positive or negative charge to the particles. The mutual repulsion of like charges provides the theoretical basis for the stabilization of emulsion particles. On the other hand, stability is also achieved through steric repulsion, which occurs because a thick layer of emulsifier is adsorbed onto the surface of the emulsion particles. When particles approach each other, the thick emulsifier layers generate repulsive forces, preventing the particles from aggregating and coalescing [29].

10.3.1 Physical Modification

Studies have revealed that the content of myofibrillar proteins in mussels is approximately 17.19%, the content of sarcoplasmic proteins is about 48.40%, and the content of stromal proteins is around 11.39%. Protein emulsifying properties depend on multiple factors, including protein molecular size, shape, amino acid composition, net charge and its distribution, spatial conformation, flexibility, and external conditions like temperature, pH, and ionic strength. These alterations can modify protein molecular structure, thereby affecting emulsifying properties [39].

10.3.1.1 Ultrasound

Ultrasonic treatment primarily utilizes the cavitation, diffusion, and homogenization effects of sound waves to cause dissociation and aggregation of protein structures, thereby altering their physicochemical and functional properties. Studies have shown that ultrasonic treatment significantly reduces the particle size of scallop protein solutions. As ultrasonic power increases, surface hydrophobicity rises significantly. Furthermore, ultrasound enhances adsorption of scallop proteins at oil droplet interfaces, increasing adsorbed protein from 35.52% to 51.43% [10]. Electrophoresis indicates that the larger aggregates in the adsorbed proteins are composed of scallop myosin. The results of reduced SDS-PAGE show that the adsorbed proteins contain a large amount of scallop myosin and two faint bands of myosin light chains. Unadsorbed proteins contain actin, tropomyosin, and three actin light chains. Confocal laser scanning microscopy (CLSM) reveals that emulsions prepared with higher-power ultrasound exhibit smaller, more uniformly dispersed oil [10].

10.3.1.2 High-Pressure Homogenization

HPH can alter the structure and functional properties of proteins. To explore whether myofibrillar proteins from mussel meat can improve the functional properties of mixed mussel isolate proteins, the impact of HPH on salt-soluble mussel myofibrillar proteins was studied. When the pressure was increased to 80 MPa, there was a similar increasing trend in protein charge [33, 40]. At 100 MPa, HPH reduced the absolute zeta potential by promoting denaturation and the formation of aggregates. This is consistent with the promotional effect of HPH on surface hydrophobicity and functionality, including foaming and emulsifying properties, which gradually strengthen with increasing pressure, reach a maximum at 80 MPa, and begin to decline at 100 MPa [33]. The shearing and stirring effects produced by homogenization cause any small part of the fluid to move at high speed relative to another part, preventing –SH and –S–S– groups from orienting and forming disulfide bonds, which prevents further aggregation of aggregates.

Within aggregates, the relatively immobilized protein molecules facilitate disulfide bond formation. This creates a hydrophobic core surrounded by outwardly oriented hydrophilic groups, mimicking the structure of naturally soluble proteins. Enhanced solubility and increased exposure of hydrophobic groups following HPH improve the foaming and emulsifying properties of mussel myofibrillar proteins. Free sulfhydryl group content increases continuously between 0 and 100 MPa, contrasting with the trend observed in mussel protein isolates. Collectively, HPH treatment at mild pressures (60–80 MPa) shows significant potential for enhancing the functional properties of mussel proteins [33].

Wu demonstrated that HPH treatment significantly reduces scallop protein particle size while increasing surface hydrophobicity and free sulfhydryl content. These results lead to an increase in the interfacial protein adsorption rate in scallop protein emulsions. This occurs because heightened surface hydrophobicity facilitates protein adsorption at oil–water interfaces, while smaller particles provide greater surface area coverage. The increase in interfacial protein content is conducive to the stability of oil droplets in the emulsion system. CLSM confirms that higher homogenization pressures yield emulsions with smaller, more uniformly dispersed oil droplets. Yu employed acid treatment to dissociate and unfold oyster proteins. Controlled enzymatic hydrolysis, HPH, and combined treatments significantly enhanced functional properties, increasing protein solubility[13]. Both emulsifying and foaming properties were significantly enhanced in acid-treated or enzymatically hydrolyzed proteins [40].

Emulsion stability is governed by interparticle potential energy interactions. The entire system is subject to both the Coulombic attraction (UA) and repulsion (UR) between particles, and the sum of these forces determines the magnitude of the potential energy (U), which illustrates the stability of the emulsion [38]. When stability is determined by the repulsive force UR (if it is electrostatic repulsion), it is the potential energy of the electrical repulsion from the surface potential; if stability is determined by the steric repulsion of steric hindrance, it is the potential energy of this repulsive force. The height of the potential energy barrier Umax serves as an indicator of the system's stability. Empirically, Yu observed that 80 MPa homogenization of mussel myofibrillar protein increased: zeta potential by 23.64 mV, emulsifying activity index by 14.99 m^2/g, emulsion stability index by 4.3 min, foaming ability by 17.3%, and foaming stability by 29.7%; while 100 MPa homogenization increased protein solubility by 7.4% (Fig. 10.9) [14].

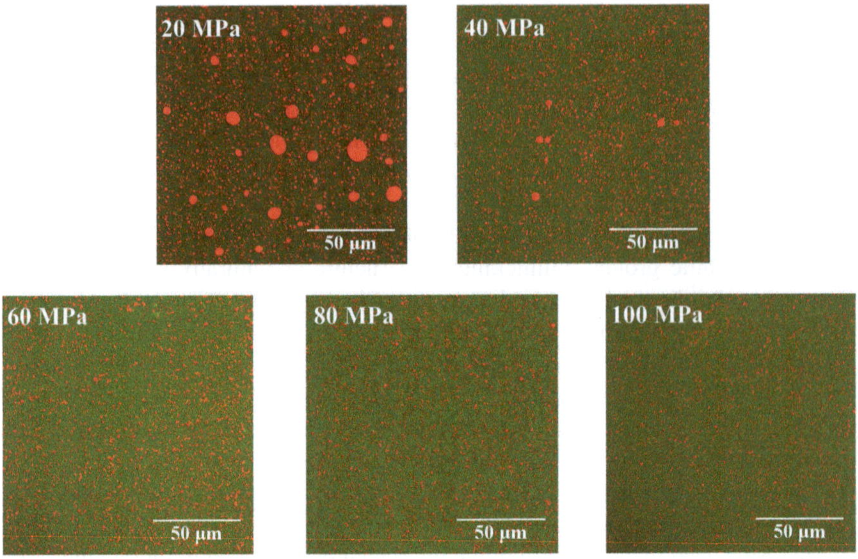

Fig. 10.9 Confocal laser scanning microscopy images of different HPH pressures of 20, 40, 60, 80, and 100 MPa. Red color represents fat droplets, and green color represents protein [4]

10.3.2 Biotechnological Modification

Enzymatic hydrolysis reduces the molecular weight of proteins, generating short peptide chains and oligopeptides. This process increases ionizable components and exposes more hydrophobic groups, thereby modifying intermolecular interactions. Guo found that heating decreased the total sulfhydryl content of oyster protein but significantly increased its surface hydrophobicity. This change resulted in an increased interfacial protein adsorption rate in oyster protein-stabilized emulsions, rising from 49.45% to 62.92% and 62.27% [15]. Further analysis by far-ultraviolet circular dichroism (CD) and fluorescence spectroscopy revealed minimal conformational changes in the tertiary structure of oyster protein. Electrophoresis analysis indicated comparable interfacial adsorption capacity for heated oyster protein. The adsorbed proteins comprised oyster actin, tropomyosin, and the three myosin light chains (LC1, LC2, LC3). Observations through CLSM and the creaming index values during storage indicated that the stability of emulsions stabilized by heated oyster protein was effectively improved [12].

10.4 Gel-Forming Ability

Protein gel formation refers to the aggregation of protein molecules, where attractive and repulsive forces are balanced, leading to highly ordered three-dimensional networks capable of retaining substantial amounts of water. The type of protein gel primarily depends on the shape of the protein molecules [41]. As gelation is dynamic, it is further modulated by environmental factors including pH, ionic strength, heating temperature, and duration. Fibrous proteins like gelatin form networks of random or helical polypeptide chains. It is reported that gelatin's gel network is formed by linear molecules creating junction zones that establish the gel network. Myofibrillar protein gels are built from three-dimensional networks formed by linear molecules connected at junction points. And globular protein thermal gels are formed by the end-to-end aggregation of protein molecules that maintain their spherical structure [41, 42]. In shellfish proteins, myosin predominates (accounting for about 43% of myofibrillar proteins), consisting of two myosin heavy chains and four myosin light chains. A portion of the two heavy chains are intertwined to form a rod-shaped α-helical structure, while another part and the four light chains form two pear-shaped heads. The overall shape resembles a bean sprout and serves as an important foundational protein for the protein gel network.

10.4.1 Physical Modification

Water plays a crucial role in protein gels. The ability to retain water is a valuable functional characteristic of protein gels. Zhang demonstrated that control myofibrillar protein (0 W) formed gels with uneven networks featuring large, irregular pores. Moderate-intensity ultrasonication (<600 W) produced denser myofibrillar protein gels with uniform networks, consistent pore sizes, and fibrous structures—particularly at 600 W. This effect may result from reduced protein particle size following ultrasonication [43]. Alternatively, decreased sulfhydryl group content and exposed hydrophobic surface groups may facilitate tighter, more uniform networks *via* disulfide bonds and hydrophobic interactions. When the ultrasonic treatment power exceeds 600 W, the gel cavities become larger and more uneven. This occurs because heat-induced gel microstructure depends critically on the relative rates of protein unfolding versus aggregation [5]. Faster aggregation relative to unfolding yields denser, more uniform microstructures, while slower aggregation produces rougher, more heterogeneous networks [43]. Therefore, after treatment with higher power ultrasonication, myofibrillar proteins undergo severe denaturation, with a large number of protein molecules unfolding and internal hydrophobicity and sulfhydryl groups exposed. When the myofibrillar protein solution is heated into a gel, the unfolding speed of the native myofibrillar protein molecules is much slower, and the aggregation speed is relatively faster, leading to a rough and uneven gel microstructure.

10.4.2 Biotechnological Modification

Enzymatic hydrolysis enables protein cross-linking or directed peptide assembly into gels. Research indicates that limited hydrolysis enhances effective hydrophobicity in certain seafood globular proteins by exposing buried polar residues, promoting aggregate formation. The promoting effect of hydrolysis on protein gels is a special property of hydrolysis products, as it is only observed under specific combinations of substrates, enzymes, and degrees of hydrolysis [44]. The solubility of hydrolysis products increases with the increase of degree of hydrolysis (DH), showing a positive correlation. Some studies believe that the solubility of protein hydrolysates is higher than that of intact proteins due to the reduction of their secondary structure, the release of smaller soluble peptides from natural proteins, and the balance of hydrophilic and hydrophobic forces of the peptides. These findings indicate that hydrolysate gel properties derive from combined protein-type and enzyme-specificity effects [40].

10.4.3 Heat

In the study of the gel characteristics of shellfish proteins, thermal processing promotes the gelation of myofibrillar proteins. To explore the relationship between the processing characteristics and muscle protein properties of the Manila clam (*Ruditapes philippinarum*), the tissue morphology, distribution characteristics of myofibrillar proteins, and their low-temperature gelation-related properties were analyzed. The results showed that the adductor muscle fibers of the Manila clam have a high degree of alignment, with striated muscles appearing as straight cylindrical shapes and smooth muscles as spiral cylindrical shapes. SDS-PAGE analysis revealed a 23-kDa differential protein in striated muscle sarcoplasmic fractions and enhanced thick filament protein solubilization. In the myofibrillar protein fraction of the smooth muscle, the typical protein Myorod was present, along with high levels of paramyosin and lower levels of myosin and actin, with actin content being close to that of the striated muscle. The solubility of the entire adductor muscle myofibrillar proteins depends on ion strength and the addition of ATP. Ca^{2+}-ATPase activity peaked at moderate ionic strength (0.30 mol/L KCl), decreasing progressively with deviations from this level. Proteins involved in cross-linking include myosin, paramyosin, and actin, with higher ionic strength leading to more significant cross-linking effects. These findings provide a reference for exploring the protein characteristics of the edible parts of economic mollusks [11].

Shellfish muscle tissue comprises both striated and smooth muscle types, featuring high paramyosin content. Adding seto scallop adductor muscle protein to silver carp muscle to create protein gels significantly improves the gel strength of the product. Research has found that the presence of paramyosin has a significant impact on the characteristics of muscle gels, with a higher content of smooth muscle forming hard and brittle gels. Studies on the thermogelling properties of salt-soluble proteins from scallop striated adductor muscle found that, compared to heating at 90 °C, the low-temperature (25 °C) gelation process plays a more important role in protein gel formation, due to the cross-linking action of transglutaminase (TGase) [40]. Fish surimi gels are formed by the dissolution of actomyosin from fish paste after salt addition, followed by protein denaturation and aggregation, leading to the formation of a three-dimensional network structure [40, 44]. The Manila clam, as an important source of aquatic protein, has been less focused on in terms of its food raw material properties. The study analyzes the composition and distribution of nitrogenous substances in the soft tissues of the Manila clam, with primary focus on myofibrillar proteins [45]. It examines the distribution characteristics of these proteins and their associated properties during low-temperature gelation—including solubility, Ca^{2+}-ATPase activity, and cross-linking characteristics under TGase action. The goal is to provide a reference for investigating the protein characteristics of the edible parts of economic mollusks [39].

10.5 Summary

Marine shellfish processing in China boasts a long history, large scale, and diverse types. Given their status as a high-protein food, regulating the properties of marine shellfish proteins during processing is particularly crucial. Altering the structure of marine shellfish proteins through physical, chemical, or biological methods to enhance their water-holding, emulsifying, and gelling properties—tailored to specific product requirements—holds significant importance. This approach is vital for diversifying marine shellfish products, boosting economic returns, and advancing related industries. The text summarizes and generalizes the methods of property regulation of marine shellfish proteins and the impact of each regulation method on protein properties, aiming to provide methods and theoretical foundations for the processing applications of marine shellfish.

References

1. Wu M, He X, Feng D, Li H, Han D, Li Q, Zhao B, Li N, Liu T, Wang J. The effect of high pressure homogenization on the structure of dual-protein and its emulsion functional properties. Foods. 2023;12(18):3358.
2. Chavan U, Mckenzie D, Shahidi F. Functional properties of protein isolates from beach pea (*Lathyrus maritimus* L.). Food Chem. 2001;74(2):177–87.
3. Wu D, Wu C, Chen H, Wang Z, Yu C, Du M. Effect of ball mill treatment on the physicochemical properties and digestibility of protein extracts generated from scallops (*Chlamys farreri*). Int J Mol Sci. 2018;19(2):531.
4. Xiong YL. Structure-function relationships of muscle proteins. In: Food proteins and their applications. CRC Press; 2017. p. 341–92.

5. Balange A, Benjakul S. Enhancement of gel strength of bigeye snapper (*Priacanthus tayenus*) surimi using oxidised phenolic compounds. Food Chem. 2009;113(1):61–70.
6. Wang Z, Chang S, Li Y, Kong L, Wu D, Qin L, Yu C, Wu C, Du M. Effects of ball milling treatment on physicochemical properties and digestibility of Pacific oyster (*Crassostrea gigas*) protein powder. Food Sci Nutr. 2018;6(6):1582–90.
7. Wu D, Tu M, Wang Z, Wu C, Yu C, Battino M, El-Seedi H, Du M. Biological and conventional food processing modifications on food proteins: structure, functionality, and bioactivity. Biotechnol Adv. 2020;40:107491.
8. Kentish S, Feng H. Applications of power ultrasound in food processing. Annu Rev Food Sci Technol. 2014;5(1):263–84.
9. Soria A, Villamiel M. Effect of ultrasound on the technological properties and bioactivity of food: a review. Trends Food Sci Technol. 2010;21(7):323–31.
10. Wu D, Wu C, Ma W, Wang Z, Yu C, Du M. Effects of ultrasound treatment on the physicochemical and emulsifying properties of proteins from scallops (*Chlamys farreri*). Food Hydrocoll. 2019;89:707–14.
11. Higuera-Barraza O, Torres-Arreola W, Ezquerra-Brauer J, Cinco-Moroyoqui F, Rodríguez Figueroa J, Marquez-Ríos E. Effect of pulsed ultrasound on the physicochemical characteristics and emulsifying properties of squid (*Dosidicus gigas*) mantle proteins. Ultrason Sonochem. 2017;38:829–34.
12. Jambrak A, Mason T, Lelas V, Herceg Z, Herceg I. Effect of ultrasound treatment on solubility and foaming properties of whey protein suspensions. J Food Eng. 2008;86(2):281–7.
13. Zhang Z, Yang Y, Zhou P, Zhang X, Wang J. Effects of high-pressure modification on conformation and gelation properties of myofibrillar protein. Food Chem. 2017;217:678–86.
14. Wu D, Wu C, Wang Z, Fan F, Chen H, Ma W, Du M. Effects of high pressure homogenize treatment on the physicochemical and emulsifying properties of proteins from scallop (*Chlamys farreri*). Food Hydrocoll. 2019;94:537–45.
15. Guo Z, Zhao F, Chen H, Tu M, Tao S, Wang Z, Wu C, He S, Du M. Heat treatments of peptides from oyster (*Crassostrea gigas*) and the impact on their digestibility and angiotensin I converting enzyme inhibitory activity. Food Sci Biotechnol. 2020;29(7):961–7.
16. Liu Z, Guo Z, Wu D, Fei X, Ei-Seedi H, Wang C. High-pressure homogenization influences the functional properties of protein from oyster (*Crassostrea gigas*). LWT-Food Sci Technol. 2021;151:112107.
17. Anthony J, Hadgis P, Milam R, Herzfeld G, Taper L, Richey S. Yields, proximate composition and mineral content of finfish and shellfish. J Food Sci. 1983;48:313–4.
18. Venugopal V, Gopakumar K. Shellfish: nutritive value, health benefits, and consumer safety. Compr Rev Food Sci Food Saf. 2017;16(6):1219–42.
19. Benson K, Galla H, Kehr N. Cell adhesion behavior in 3D hydrogel scaffolds functionalized with D- or L-Aminoacids. Macromol Biosci. 2014;14(6):793–8.
20. Veldkamp K, Tubergen P, Swartz M, DeVries J, Tatko C. Zinc binding with l-dopa peptides. Inorg Chim Acta. 2017;461:120–6.
21. Xiong H. ZnO nanoparticles applied to bioimaging and drug delivery. Adv Mater. 2013;25(37):5329–35.
22. Liu X, Zheng C, Luo X, Wang X, Jiang H. Recent advances of collagen-based biomaterials: multi-hierarchical structure, modification and biomedical applications. Mater Sci Eng. 2019;99:1509–22.
23. Han J, Shang W, Yan J, Du Y, McClements D, Xiao H, Wu H, Zhu B. Protection of β-carotene from chemical degradation in emulsion-based delivery systems using scallop (*Patinopecten yessoensis*) gonad protein isolates. Food Bioprocess Technol. 2020;13(4):680–92.
24. Mannheim A, Cheryan M. Enzyme–modified proteins from corn gluten meal: preparation and functional properties. J Am Oil Chem Soc. 1992;69(12):1163.
25. Yuan B, Ren J, Zhao M, Luo D, Gu L. Effects of limited enzymatic hydrolysis with pepsin and high-pressure homogenization on the functional properties of soybean protein isolate. LWT Food Sci Technol. 2012;46(2):453–9.

26. Tavano O. Protein hydrolysis using proteases: an important tool for food biotechnology. J Mol Catal B Enzym. 2013;90:1–11.
27. Zhang Z, Zhou F, Liu X, Zhao M. Particulate nanocomposite from oyster (*Crassostrea rivularis*) hydrolysates *via* zinc chelation improves zinc solubility and peptide activity. Food Chem. 2018;258:269–77.
28. Martínez-Fernández E, Acosta-Salmón H, Southgate P. The nutritional value of seven species of tropical microalgae for black-lip pearl oyster (*Pinctada margaritifera, L.*) larvae. Aquaculture. 2006;257(1–4):491–503.
29. Yu C, Wu F, Cha Y, Zou H, Bao J, Xu R, Du M. Effects of high-pressure homogenization on functional properties and structure of mussel (*Mytilus edulis*) myofibrillar proteins. Int J Biol Macromol. 2018;118:741–6.
30. Wu D, Wu C, Tu M, Yu C, Du M. Identification and analysis of bioactive peptides from scallops (*Chlamys farreri*) protein by simulated gastrointestinal digestion. J Food Process Preserv. 2018;42(9):e13760.
31. He S, Zhang Y, Sun H, Du M, Qiu J, Tang M, Sun X, Zhu B. Antioxidative peptides from proteolytic hydrolysates of false abalone (*Volutharpa ampullacea perryi*): characterization, identification, and molecular docking. Mar Drugs. 2019;17(2):116.
32. Qiao M, Tu M, Wang Z, Mao F, Chen H, Qin L, Du M. Identification and antithrombotic activity of peptides from blue mussel (*Mytilus edulis*) protein. Int J Mol Sci. 2018;19(1):138.
33. Yu C, Cha Y, Wu F, Xu X, Du M. Effects of limited hydrolysis and high-pressure homogenization on functional properties of oyster protein isolates. Molecules. 2018;23(4):729.
34. Qiao M, Tu M, Chen H, Mao F, Yu C, Du M. Identification and in Silico prediction of anticoagulant peptides from the enzymatic hydrolysates of *Mytilus edulis* proteins. Int J Mol Sci. 2018;19(7):2100.
35. Wali A, Ma H, Shahnawaz M, Hayat K, Xiaong J, Jing L. Impact of power ultrasound on antihypertensive activity, functional properties, and thermal stability of rapeseed protein hydrolysates. J Chem. 2017;2017:1–11.
36. Jin W, Wu H, Zhu B, Ran X. Functional properties of gelation-like protein hydrolysates from scallop (*Patinopecten yessoensis*) male gonad. Eur Food Res Technol. 2012;234(5):863–72.
37. Mao F, Shi P, Chen H, Song L, Wang Z, Wu C, Du M. Beneficial effects of polysaccharides on the solubility of Mytilus edulis enzymatic hydrolysates. Food Chem. 2018;254:103–8.
38. Torres O, Murray B, Sarkar A. Emulsion microgel particles: novel encapsulation strategy for lipophilic molecules. Trends Food Sci Technol. 2016;55:98–108.
39. Yu C, Wu F, Cha F, Qin Y, Du M. Effects of ultrasound on structure and functional properties of mussel (*Mytilus edulis*) protein isolates. J Food Process Preserv. 2018;42(8):e13690.
40. Yu C, Cha Y, Wu F, Xu X, Qin Y, Li X, Du M. Effects of high-pressure homogenisation on structural and functional properties of mussel (*Mytilus edulis*) protein isolate. Int J Food Sci Technol. 2018;53(5):1157–65.
41. Zhang Z, Regenstein J, Zhou P, Yang Y. Effects of high intensity ultrasound modification on physicochemical property and water in myofibrillar protein gel. Ultrason Sonochem. 2017;34:960–7.
42. Takahashi K, Kurose K, Okazaki E, Osako K. Effect of various protease inhibitors on heat-induced myofibrillar protein degradation and gel-forming ability of red tilefish (*Branchiostegus japonicus*) meat. LWT Food Sci Technol. 2016;68:717–23.
43. Xiong X, He B, Jiang D, Dong X, Koosis A, Yu C, Qi H. Postmortem biochemical and textural changes in the *Patinopecten yessoensis* adductor muscle (PYAM) during iced storage. Int J Food Prop. 2019;22(1):1024–34.
44. Yu Y, Fan F, Wu D, Yu C, Wang Z, Du M. Antioxidant and ACE inhibitory activity of enzymatic hydrolysates from *Ruditapes philippinarum*. Molecules. 2018;23(5):1189.
45. Cha Y, Wu F, Zou H, Shi X, Zhao Y, Bao J, Du M, Yu C. High-pressure homogenization pretreatment improved functional properties of oyster protein isolate hydrolysates. Molecules. 2018;23(12):3344.

Chapter 11
Sensitization and Control of Marine Shellfish Proteins

Ming Du, Hui Chen, Zhaorui Li, and Shaoyun Wang

Abstract This chapter examines the sensitization potential of marine shellfish proteins and strategies for managing them. Initially, the mechanisms of food-allergic reactions, including IgE-mediated rapid and delayed hypersensitivity reactions, are presented. Subsequently, this section addresses the epidemiology and clinical manifestations of allergic reactions to marine shellfish and provides an overview of the most common allergenic proteins found in shellfish, including promyosin, arginine kinase, and myosin light chain, along with a description of their biological properties. Furthermore, a range of methodologies for the detection of shellfish allergens are presented, including ELISA, immunoblotting, biosensors, mass spectrometry, and others. Finally, this section will discuss the allergenicity control methods that can be applied to marine shellfish proteins. These include thermal processing treatments, biochemical methods (e.g., glycosylation, enzymolysis, and fermentation), and novel processing methods (e.g., ultrasound, irradiation, and pulsed UV).

Keywords Marine shellfish proteins · Allergenicity · Mechanism of allergic reactions · Allergen detection methods · Allergen control methods

Food allergy represents an abnormal immune response to food proteins, triggering adverse clinical symptoms. These disorders encompass potentially fatal acute reactions along with chronic conditions primarily involving the skin and gastrointestinal tract. Food allergies are classified into (1) IgE-mediated reactions, (2) mixed IgE- and non-IgE-mediated disorders, and (3) non-IgE-mediated disorders. IgE-mediated reactions manifest as immediate gastrointestinal hypersensitivity or oral allergy

M. Du (✉)
College of Food Science and Engineering, Dalian Ocean University, Dalian, China

H. Chen
Food Science and Engineering, Zhejiang University of Technology, Zhejiang, China

Z. Li
Food Science and Engineering, Dalian Polytechnic University, Dalian, China

S. Wang
Biological Science and Engineering, Fuzhou University, Fuzhou, China

M. Du, S. Cheng (eds.), *Bioactive Proteins and Peptides from Marine Shellfish*,
https://doi.org/10.1007/978-981-95-3937-6_11

syndrome. Immediate hypersensitivity syndromes, which typically manifest as disturbances in the skin, respiratory, gastrointestinal, or systemic reactions, are known as anaphylactic reactions. In general, the diagnosis of a person with food allergy can be confirmed by serum-specific IgE antibody measurements combined with skin tests to confirm the pattern of IgE-mediated reactions [1].

Oral allergy syndrome (OAS) represents an IgE-mediated allergic reaction triggered by contact with food antigens on mucosal surfaces. Although OAS can affect other organ systems, it most commonly presents with symptoms within minutes to hours after ingestion. Non-IgE-mediated gastrointestinal disorders are typically classified as dietary protein enteropathies, with dietary protein colitis and celiac disease representing the most prevalent forms. These conditions are commonly triggered by milk or soy proteins, causing variable intestinal damage characterized by nonspecific villous atrophy and mucosal inflammation. Mixed IgE- and non-IgE-mediated diseases include eosinophilic gastroenteritis, eosinophilic proctocolitis, eosinophilic gastroenteritis, and eosinophilic esophagitis. These diseases are distinguished by an infiltration of the gastrointestinal tract by eosinophils in the absence of other inflammatory cells [1].

11.1 Mechanisms of Food-Allergic Reactions

Food proteins recognized by IgE as triggers for adverse reactions constitute allergens. These allergens are predominantly proteins or glycoproteins with molecular weights typically ranging from 5 to 70 kDa. In the case of rapid-onset hypersensitivity reactions, the onset of symptoms occurs within minutes to an hour after ingestion of the allergen. This is accompanied by an abnormal response of the humoral immune system, namely the formation of allergen-specific IgE antibodies [2]. Delayed hypersensitivity reactions manifest more than 24 h after exposure, mediated primarily by antigen-specific T cell responses. Hypersensitivity reactions progress through two key phases: (1) sensitization phase: initial exposure leading to IgE production and (2) effector phase: IgE-triggered inflammatory cascade. Figure 11.1 illustrates this pathophysiological process.

To initiate an allergic response, food allergens must initially contact gastrointestinal mucosal surfaces. Upon initial exposure, allergens are taken up by antigen-presenting cells (APCs), specifically intestinal lamina propria dendritic cells. Allergens are internalized by dendritic cells through receptor-mediated endocytosis, macrocytosis, or merging with microvesicles shed from the surface of neighboring cells, as well as interactions with nanovesicles or exosomes [2]. These sensitizers can be identified through the use of ubiquitin, a highly conserved protein comprising 76 residues present in all eukaryotic organisms. Ubiquitin conjugation marks allergens for proteasomal degradation. Ubiquitinated allergens undergo proteasomal processing into peptide fragments. The degraded peptide fragments are then presented by major histocompatibility complex class II (MHC-II) and recognized by naïve CD4+ T cells.

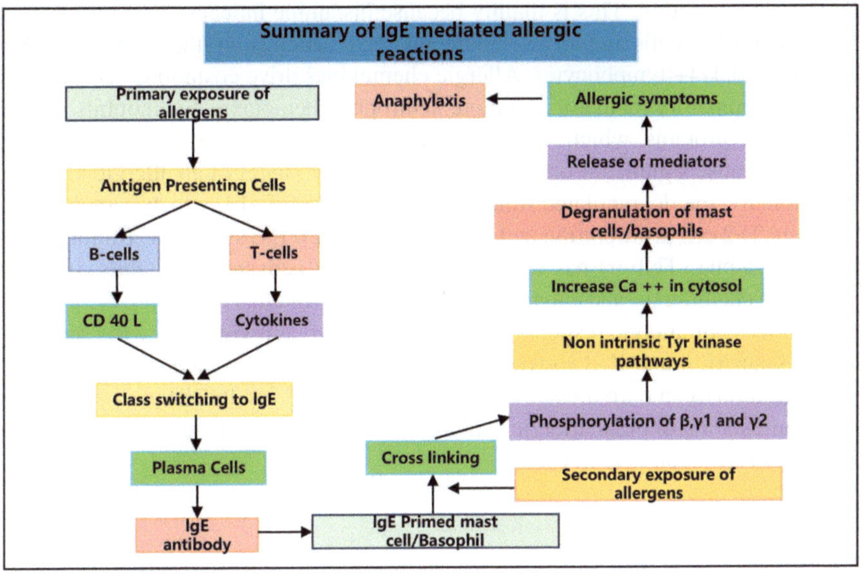

Fig. 11.1 Summary of the process of food-allergic reactions

CD4+ T helper (Th) cells are classified into Th1 and Th2 subsets based on their cytokine profiles. Interleukin-4 (IL-4) drives the differentiation of naive CD4+ T cells into Th2 cells. Differentiated Th2 cells can secrete the cytokines IL-4 and IL-13, which induce their class conversion to IgE. Furthermore, the pivotal function of IgE in both the initial and subsequent phases of allergic inflammation has been established. B cell IgE synthesis requires two T cell-derived signals: (1) IL-4 and IL-13 signaling and (2) CD40-CD40L engagement between B cells and Th2 cells [3]. The activation of IgE synthesis by B cells requires the implementation of signal transduction by T cells. Both signals are mediated by the activation of Janus family tyrosine kinases 1 and 3, which ultimately leads to the phosphorylation of signal transducers and activators of transcription 6.

During sensitization, IgE-producing B cells release IgE into systemic circulation, which binds to high-affinity receptors on tissue-resident mast cells and basophils. Allergen cross-linking of receptor-bound IgE triggers degranulation, releasing preformed mediators like histamine, prostaglandins, and leukotrienes [4, 5]. Mast cell activation induces (1) immediate release of preformed mediators (histamine, tryptase) and (2) de novo synthesis of lipid mediators and cytokines. Histamine is an organic nitrogenous compound that is produced from histidine in the presence of the enzyme decarboxylase. Mast cells of many tissues, especially the skin, lungs, and intestinal mucosa, contain significant quantities of histamine. The release of histamine can be triggered by tissue damage or the onset of inflammatory and allergic reactions. The primary effects of histamine are mediated by two distinct receptors: H1 and H2. Upon binding to these receptors, histamine causes the contraction of airway and gastrointestinal smooth muscle, increased vascular permeability and vasodilation, enhanced mucus production, itching, cutaneous vasodilatation, and gastric acid secretion. This is mainly because histamine induces the production of IL-16 by CD8 + cells and airway epithelial cells, which is an important early chemokine for CD4+ lymphocytes. Allergic chemokines drive eosinophil recruitment, while inflammatory mediators promote neutrophil chemotaxis. Eosinophils release major basic proteins, which, when combined with the effects of activated neutrophils, can cause significant tissue damage in the later stages of an allergic reaction. Additionally, the degranulated fluid contains IL-4 and IL-13, which stimulate and maintain Th2 cell proliferation and shift B cells toward IgE synthesis. Tumor necrosis factor-alpha (TNF-α) has been demonstrated to activate neutrophils, increase monocyte chemotaxis, and enhance T-cell production of other cytokines. Subsequent to the release of allergic response mediators, effector cells commence the secretion of cytokines IL-4 and IL-13 several hours later. The released mediators may result in the dilation of smooth muscles, the rupture of capillaries, localized swelling, and the manifestation of other allergic symptoms. Severe cases may progress to anaphylaxis, with rare fatal outcomes.

11.2 Allergic Reactions

11.2.1 Epidemiology of Marine Shellfish Allergy

Globally, 3.5–4.0% of the population experiences food allergies. Among these, shellfish allergies represent a predominant subset, with potential for severe manifestations. Shellfish allergy prevalence ranges from 0.5% to 2.5% worldwide, showing significant variation based on consumption patterns, age, and geographic region [2]. The prevalence of occupational contact dermatitis due to shellfish ranges from 3% to 11%. Asian populations demonstrate higher shellfish allergy rates than Western cohorts. A study of children residing in Singapore revealed a higher prevalence of allergies among local children compared to national averages. Among children aged 4–6 years, 1.19% exhibited allergic symptoms, while 0.55% of the same age group demonstrated allergic tendencies. Among children aged 14–16 years, the prevalence was 5.23% and 0.96%, respectively.

While predominantly affecting adults and older children, shellfish allergies may develop at any age, including to previously tolerated foods. It is not uncommon for individuals with a shellfish allergy to retain this sensitivity throughout their lifetime. The prevalence of shellfish allergies is geographically widespread, largely due to the ready availability of these foods. In individuals who have been occupationally sensitized to shellfish products, exposure to these products can trigger sensitization reactions *via* the respiratory or dermal routes. Mollusk allergy prevalence is highest in France, Spain, Hong Kong (China), and Singapore, but lower in the United Kingdom and Germany. Mainland China lacks comprehensive epidemiologic data, thus excluded from current statistics. The prevalence of shellfish allergy in Hong Kong is approximately 37.8%. Additionally, it has been documented that mollusks are responsible for approximately 5.6% and 11.7% of severe reactions in France, and 36% of allergic reactions in Singapore are triggered by molluscan exposure.

11.2.2 Manifestations of Allergic Reactions

Seafood is a significant component of a healthy diet and plays an important role in human nutrition and health. China, the United States, and Japan represent the three largest consumer markets for seafood globally. As consumption of seafood has increased, adverse health events have become more prevalent among consumers and those engaged in the processing of seafood. The primary adverse reactions to shellfish are attributable to immune system-mediated reactions (allergies) and nonimmune reactions. Certain shellfish components provoke allergy-like symptoms through nonimmunologic mechanisms, mimicking true IgE-mediated reactions [6]. The majority of shellfish are not allergenic. Given the similarity in clinical reactions among individuals, it is of paramount importance to distinguish adverse reactions from true shellfish allergies and comprehend the molecular nature of the sensitizer and the underlying mechanisms of the allergic reaction.

A shellfish allergy is a subtype of seafood allergy, characterized by an adverse immune reaction to shellfish consumption. This hypersensitivity triggers an exaggerated immune response that manifests in severe physical symptoms. Symptoms range from itching and swelling of the mouth and throat (oral allergy syndrome) to potentially life-threatening anaphylaxis. Reactions can occur not only after ingestion by a sensitized individual, but also through inhalation of cooking vapors. It is estimated that 75% of individuals with an allergic reaction to one type of crustacean (e.g., shrimp, lobster, crayfish, or crab) are also allergic to other types of crustaceans [7]. Given the similarity in the proteins present in crustaceans and mollusks (including promyosin, paramyosin, and arginine kinase), it is plausible that individuals may exhibit a similar allergic response to both types of foods [8–10].

11.3 Sensitization and Evaluation

11.3.1 Biological Characterization

Proto-myosin was the initial sensitizer identified in shellfish, followed by the discovery of other sensitizer proteins, including arginine kinase (AK), myosin light chain (MLC), and calcium-binding sarcoplasmic protein (SCP) [11]. The following section provides an overview of the allergenic proteins present in various shellfish species and their associated biological properties.

1. Protomyosin

The first recognition of protomyosin as a heat-stable, soluble sensitizer in crustaceans occurred in 1981. It consists of 281 amino acids with a molecular weight of 38–41 kDa. Protomyosin is expressed in both muscle and nonmuscle cells of shellfish [12, 13]. In muscle tissue, it regulates contraction by mediating troponin-actin interactions. Protomyosin is a coiled-coil protein constituted by two parallel α-helices, each containing two sets of seven alternate binding sites on actin. The troponin-protomyosin complex serves to regulate the Ca^{2+}-dependent interaction between actin and myosin. Protomyosin molecules form a continuous chain along actin filaments through a process known as "head-to-tail polymerization." Each protomyosin molecule binds to seven actin monomers *via* Tns I, T, and C (calcium-binding subunits). In non-myocytes, protomyosin fulfills the function of providing mechanical support for the transport of cytoplasmic membranes and other molecules. Subsequently, protomyosin, to which it belongs, was identified in various shrimp, lobster, and crab species, serving as a primary sensitizer in mollusks such as abalone, conch, horned turban, clams, razor shells, mussels, oysters, scallops, octopus, and squid [14]. Invertebrate protomyosin is a pan-sensitizer, whereas vertebrate protomyosin is typically not sensitizing.

In recent years, informatics-based methods have been employed for the study of antigenic epitopes of protomyosin. In summary, potential epitopes can be predicted by a computerized system based on a combination of amino acid properties (hydrophobicity, flexibility, accessibility, exposed surface, polarity, and antigenicity). The calculated potential epitopes can then be synthesized and validated by inhibition assays. The antigenic epitope peptides obtained by this computer-based approach can be screened for sequences that react in serum.

2. Arginine Kinase

AK is a phospho-ATP phosphotransferase generally found in invertebrates and plays a crucial role in energy metabolism [12]. As is the case with the majority of enzymes, AK is an intolerant sensitizer. It has regulatory and transport properties and is abundant not only in crustacean muscle but also plays a crucial role in invertebrate metabolism, catalyzing the reversible transfer of high-energy phosphates from arginine phosphate to ADP to form ATP. Crustacean arginine kinase has similar metabolic roles to vertebrate creatinine kinase. Additionally, arginine kinase is a pan-allergen in invertebrate shellfish, shrimps, and crabs, similar to protomyosin.

Penm 2 (MW = 40 kDa) is an allergenic protein with arginine kinase activity that was identified from shrimp by two-dimensional immunoblotting and MALDI-TOF methods.

This sensitizer was identified in 94% of allergic patients. AK has also been identified in various mollusks, showing high sequence homology across species. Studies have demonstrated that oyster AK exists in seven antigenic epitopes and that the allergen is more unstable at temperatures higher than 40 °C or at pH $\leq$ 5.0.

3. Myosin Light Chain

MLCs are muscle proteins with a molecular weight of 20 kDa and are a novel marine sensitizer. Myosins constitute a large superfamily of muscle proteins that are involved in muscle contraction and hydrolysis of ADP along actin filaments [15]. During muscle contraction, intracellular calcium ion concentrations rise. These ions bind troponin C, inducing conformational change. This, in turn, causes the release of protropomyosin and the exposure of the actin-binding site [16]. The actin-troponin binding complex is influenced by the phosphorylation of myosin light chains, which results in conformational alterations in myosin, thereby enabling muscle contraction. Although the original myosin is considered the primary sensitizer, some patients exhibit sensitivity to MLCs. The molecular weight and isoelectric point of the protein in question are similar to those of matrix calcium-binding proteins, which makes it challenging to distinguish between the two. Additionally, it was observed that IgE binding to boiled myosin light chains exhibited a stronger affinity in adults compared to children, who demonstrated a higher intensity of recognition for MLCs in raw extracts.

4. Paramyosin

Paramyosin is a 103 kDa cross-reactive muscle protein that is found in a variety of invertebrates. In mollusks, paramyosin plays a role in a "trapping" mechanism that conserves energy, maintaining muscle contraction with minimal expenditure [17]. Der p 11, the allergen of the house dust mite, exhibits substantial homology, with approximately 89% sequence similarity, to the paramecium of mollusks such as the Mediterranean black mussel (*Myt g* PM), the Pacific abalone (*Hal d* PM), the horned turban snail turbo (*Tur c* PM), and the common octopus (*Oct v* PM).

5. Matrix Calcium-Binding Protein

Matrix calcium-binding proteins are acidic calcium-binding proteins found in the cytoplasm with a molecular weight of 20–22 kDa. They are immunorecognized in approximately 50% of patients. Matrix calcium-binding proteins are polypeptide chain dimers with three calcium-binding sites, designated αα, αβ, and ββ. It is hypothesized that matrix calcium-binding proteins play a functional role analogous to that of small proteins in promoting muscle relaxation, whereby Ca^{2+} is transferred from myofibrils to the sarcoplasmic reticulum. Matrix calcium-binding protein is a glycoprotein sensitizer containing 4.9% carbohydrate, as determined by the phenol-sulfuric acid method. Matrix calcium-binding protein exhibits resistance to heat, acid, and alkali treatment and stability in buffers with a pH range of 1–11. However, it can be completely digested within an hour. Matrix calcium-binding protein is a polymorphic sensitizer with three isoforms (matrix calcium-binding protein-I, matrix calcium-binding protein-II, and matrix calcium-binding protein-III) with pIs of 5.05, 4.90, and 4.75, respectively. All three isoforms can bind to IgE [18].

6. Troponin C

Troponin is comprised of three subunits: troponin C, which binds to Ca^{2+}, troponin I, which binds to actin and inhibits actin-myosin interactions, and troponin T, which binds to protropomyosin.

Troponin C is a member of a family of homologous proteins that includes calmodulin, myosin light chain, and small serotonin [19]. A sequence analysis revealed that troponin has four calcium-binding regions (I–IV), each of which contains a pair of helices located on either side of the 12-residue calcium-binding site. Crystallographic studies demonstrated the existence of two discrete regions, connected by a central helix, each with two calcium-binding sites. Two high-affinity sites (III and IV) and two low-affinity sites (I and II) are responsible for muscle contraction; however, only regions II and IV are biologically functional.

7. Additional Sensitizing Proteins

Other minor sensitizers have been described, including alpha-actinin with a molecular weight of 31–42 kDa, which is recognized by 22% of patients; smooth endoplasmic reticulum Ca^{2+}-ATPase with a molecular weight of 113 kDa; and glyceraldehyde-3-phosphate dehydrogenase with a molecular weight of 37 kDa.

11.3.2 Methods for the Detection

Food allergies primarily involve IgE-mediated responses to specific food antigens. Even trace amounts of allergens can trigger a strong reaction in highly sensitive individuals. These reactions may present as urticaria and atopic dermatitis on the skin. They can also manifest as rhinitis and asthma in the respiratory system, or edema and hypotension in the circulatory system. In severe cases, they may even lead to life-threatening acute responses like IgE-mediated anaphylaxis. The food industry and food manufacturers ensure that food allergens are clearly labeled and employ a variety of methods for the detection of food allergens. These analytical methods must demonstrate high specificity, sensitivity, and matrix interference resistance. These methods are capable of targeting both allergenic proteins and allergenic markers, which may be peptides or gene fragments. Protein-based methods, which rely heavily on immunological techniques, are a widely utilized approach for identifying the sensitizer itself. Protein-based methods include enzyme-linked immunosorbent assays (ELISA), immunoblotting, mass spectrometry, and biosensors. DNA-based methods include endpoint quantitative PCR, real-time PCR, and PCR-ELISA [20].

1. ELISA

ELISA has been developed as a safer alternative to radioimmunoassay and has demonstrated significant potential in biochemical and biomedical applications as early as the 1980s. As the current gold standard for food allergen detection, ELISA offers straightforward implementation, matrix versatility, and high protein sensitivity. Its high sensitivity, low cost, and operational simplicity make ELISA the industry standard for monitoring allergen contamination. Concurrently, the high potential of ELISA for standardization and automation has facilitated the fulfillment of the demand for a considerable number of samples. ELISA is primarily classified into two main categories: competitive (direct) and sandwich methods. In competitive ELISA, the food allergen is immobilized on a plate and competes with the allergen in the sample for binding to an enzyme-labeled primary antibody. In sandwich ELISA, in contrast, the allergen is captured by two antibodies forming a sandwich. The allergen is captured by these antibodies, the primary antibody on the immobilized phase captures the allergen. And then it is further detected by the allergen-specific secondary antibody labeled by an enzyme or other marker molecule (e.g., biotin).

2. Immunoblotting
   Immunoblotting methods used for allergen analysis include protein blotting and spot blotting. Western blotting is a technique that separates proteins by molecular weight using polyacrylamide gel electrophoresis (PAGE). The separated proteins are then transferred to a membrane (e.g., PVDF or nitrocellulose) for antibody detection. A key disadvantage of Western blotting is that proteins are typically analyzed in a denatured state. This can lead to the loss of conformational epitopes due to disruption of the protein's native structure. Moreover, denaturation may expose novel IgE-binding epitopes normally concealed within the native protein structure. Additionally, since separation relies on molecular weight, proteins falling outside the effective resolution range of the gel or membrane may not be adequately separated. Western blotting offers the advantage of enabling separate analysis of individual protein bands, facilitating the identification of changes in specific allergens. The technique is also relatively rapid, straightforward, and cost-effective. In dot blot analysis, the sample is directly adsorbed onto a membrane (typically nitrocellulose) and probed with antibodies for detection. This method avoids denaturing conditions, thereby preserving native conformational epitopes. Unlike Western blotting, which separates proteins by molecular weight, dot blotting enables analysis of the immunoreactivity of the entire sample. Furthermore, individual isolated proteins can also be analyzed using this technique.

3. Biosensors
   Biosensors represent a novel approach to the detection of allergenic components in foodstuffs. While capable of detecting DNA or protein analytes, biosensors are currently used primarily for protein detection. The principal advantages of this approach are the relatively short analysis time and the potential for automation. Optical biosensors also facilitate the development of direct and sandwich immunoassays for the detection of proteins in a range of food samples, including milk, eggs, hazelnuts, peanuts, shellfish, and sesame seeds. Affinity-purified polyclonal antibodies are immobilized on the biosensor chip. Food samples are then injected, and bound allergenic proteins are detected through resonance angular shifts. Incorporating a secondary antibody in the sandwich format overcomes matrix effects while improving sensitivity and selectivity. Biosensors using surface plasmon resonance or biofilm interference detect food allergens at levels of 1–12.5 μg/g in food matrices, demonstrating sensitivity comparable to immunoassays like ELISA.

4. Mass Spectrometry
   Mass spectrometry is now widely employed for protein analysis. The application of proteomic methods in the analysis of food allergens is called "allergen genomics." Mass spectrometry serves two primary roles in allergen proteomics: (1) elucidating the structural and functional characteristics of food allergens, and (2) developing reliable quantitative methods for detecting allergens across a range of concentrations, including trace levels. Mass spectrometry enables rapid, accurate protein analysis with high sensitivity, specificity, and reproducibility. Matrix-assisted laser desorption ionization and electrospray ionization have been the most

widely used ionization techniques for biomolecular analysis since their introduction in the late 1980s. Mass spectrometry can determine the molecular mass of proteins and peptides, and characterize structural details including amino acid sequences, post-translational modifications, and process-induced modifications.

In the context of allergen detection and identification, mass spectrometry is frequently employed in conjunction with separation techniques, including unidirectional electrophoresis one-dimensional polyacrylamide gel electrophoresis (1D-PAGE) and bidirectional electrophoresis two-dimensional polyacrylamide gel electrophoresis (2D-PAGE), as well as liquid chromatography (LC). 2D-PAGE is a reliable and efficient method for separating complex protein mixtures. In the first dimension (isoelectric focusing), proteins separate according to isoelectric point (pI), while in the second dimension (SDS-PAGE), they separate by molecular weight. Following visualization, the protein spots excised from the gel were subjected to in situ digestion with protease and subsequently analyzed by MS or MS/MS for identification purposes. Protein identification by peptide mass fingerprinting (PMF) enables a comparison of the mass spectrometry-identified molecular weights with the theoretically expected peptide mass of each entry in the database.

Mass spectrometric analysis of peptides using techniques like MALDI-TOF/TOF or ESI-MS/MS provides detailed structural information about amino acid sequences. This enables highly specific and high-resolution identification. The primary process of the LC-MS method is the hydrolysis of allergenic proteins extracted from food. This is typically performed with trypsin, which selectively cleaves proteins at the C-terminus of specific residues. The resulting peptide mixture is separated *via* liquid chromatography, which exploits differential affinities between peptides, the stationary phase, and the mobile phase. Peptides are then ionized by electrospray and analyzed by mass spectrometry. A variety of mass spectrometry techniques have been employed for the quantification of food allergens. Triple quadrupole (QQQ) instruments operating in multiple reaction monitoring (MRM) mode are most common, detecting characteristic fragment ions generated through collision-induced dissociation (CID) of selected precursors. Furthermore, mass spectrometry analysis modes such as full-scan mode, multiple ion monitoring (MIM), and selected ion monitoring (SIM) are also available. Moreover, quadrupole time-of-flight (Q-TOF) and quadrupole ion trap (Q-IT) are frequently employed techniques for semiquantitative proteomics. Korte developed a mass spectrometry method in MRM mode for the detection of enzymatically cleaved peptides contaminated with shrimp and lobster sensitization in complex food matrices at concentrations below 0.1% [21].

5. Endpoint Quantitative PCR

In endpoint quantitative PCR, the quantity of PCR product reflects the quantity of the target sequence in the sample. For the quantitative analysis of DNA target sequences, the use of three primer fragments (comprising two sense strands and one antisense strand) is recommended.

This pair of short primer fragments can recognize the DNA target sequence signature of a given allergen source for PCR amplification. The remaining primer fragment is employed as a probe for the detection of the specific PCR amplification product. In this process, the key factors for the attainment of quantitative results include, for instance, the quantity of Mg^{2+}, the number of positive and negative primers, dNTPs, and the DNA polymerase utilized for PCR. Furthermore, it is essential to ascertain the PCR amplification conditions, which are contingent upon the quantity of DNA and the number of amplification cycles. The logarithm of the amount of DNA is linearly related to the logarithm of the gene amplification product. This relationship is valid within a certain range, which depends on the amount of starting nucleic acid and the number of cycles of PCR. In a previous study, Taguchi employed an endpoint PCR method to identify the DNA-sensitizing components of shrimp and crab [22]. The PCR method was able to detect 5 pg of DNA from both the target species and 50 ng of genomic DNA in the induced food sample.

6. Real-Time Quantitative PCR

Real-time quantitative PCR (qPCR) is considered the gold standard for DNA and RNA analysis and is widely used for accurate quantification of food allergens. This technique analyzes target nucleic acids qualitatively and quantitatively by monitoring fluorescence signals generated during amplification of target-specific DNA sequences. For food analysis, qPCR typically uses fluorescent probes or DNA-binding dyes to detect amplification signals. The nonspecific dye SYBR Green binds double-stranded DNA (dsDNA), exhibiting significantly enhanced fluorescence upon binding. As the PCR products of specific DNA fragments are lengthened, the fluorescence intensity increases in relation to the amount of PCR product produced per double-stranded DNA (dsDNA), including nonspecific products such as primer dimers. The SYBR Green dye is a more cost-effective alternative to fluorescent probe-based analysis methods. One disadvantage of qPCR is that it may yield false-negative results due to the presence of impurities and other inhibitors in the DNA extracted from food samples. At present, conventional real-time fluorescent quantitative PCR techniques are available for the detection and quantification of crustacean allergens in complex food matrices. Eischeid developed a real-time PCR method using a fluorescent probe for the detection of allergens in lobster [23]. However, the method has been rarely reported for allergen detection in shellfish.

7. PCR-ELISA

PCR-ELISA is a technique that can be used to detect specific DNA sequences in a wide range of PCR products. This method provides a cost-effective alternative for quantifying specific amplicons and enables semi-quantitative analysis of food allergens. It achieves high sensitivity for trace DNA detection in complex food matrices. The concentration of the target DNA fragment is positively correlated with the depth of coloration of the enzyme–substrate reaction. Furthermore, the combination of ELISA analysis with conventional PCR ensures the sequence specificity of the target DNA amplification products in the sample. In this approach, the PCR product is immobilized on a solid phase. Following denaturation of the double-stranded DNA, a sequence-specific fluorescein isothiocyanate (FITC)-labeled DNA hybridization probe is introduced.

11.4 Allergen Control Methods

Currently, no reliable methods exist to prevent or cure food allergies; strict allergen avoidance remains the primary safety measure. Consequently, reducing allergens through food processing offers a viable mitigation strategy. While most allergenic epitopes exhibit partial resistance to processing, substantial evidence confirms that targeted methods can significantly alter allergenicity. In the field of food processing, a variety of methods, including physical, chemical, enzymatic, and fermentation techniques, have the potential to alter allergenic activity [24, 25]. Proteins are one of the main components of food, important nutrients, and a major allergen category in the daily diet. Food processing methods can cause changes in the spatial structure and physicochemical properties of protein macromolecules, thereby destroying the allergenic epitopes of proteins. Commonly used food processing methods to reduce allergenicity can be mainly categorized into thermal, biochemical, and novel processing methods.

11.4.1 Thermal Processing

Foods are usually heated within the two temperature ranges of pasteurization and sterilization. The impact of thermal processing on the allergenicity of allergenic components present in certain foodstuffs is frequently overlooked. Heating can either reduce allergenicity or enhance it by altering the original protein structure. The stability of a protein is contingent upon its structural form, which is largely dependent on hydrogen bonding, disulfide bonding, electrostatic, and hydrophobic interactions. Upon heating, proteins undergo progressive denaturation that intensifies with rising temperature. The molecular bonds that hold the protein allergenic structure together adjust themselves when heated, and heating breaks the balanced interaction bonds and structural adjustments occur. Heat exposure triggers reorientation of internally buried hydrophobic groups toward solvent-exposed positions. Proteins tend to start denaturing at around 50–60 °C, with changes in their tertiary structure influenced by their stability, molecular size, and molecular weight, leading to the eventual complete denaturation of the protein as the temperature continues to rise. Additionally, temperature-induced chemical reactions between proteins and other food components result in the formation and discoloration of undesired substances. This includes the Maillard reaction between amino acids and reducing sugars.

1. Hygrothermal Processing

   The utilization of water for the purpose of heating food is regarded as "hygrothermal processing." In cherries, specific Bet v1-homologous epitopes (e.g., cross-reactive epitope-2) undergo conformational changes during moist-heat processing [26]. Mal d 2, a homologue of apple Bet v 1, can also lose its structure when heated to 363 K, and a small fraction of the unexpanded structure is structurally restored when cooled back to 293 K [27]. Api g 1, which is also homologous to Bet v 1, a major celery allergen, is able to retain its allergenicity because it restores most of the original structure of the molecule [28]. Furthermore, the thermal stability of allergenic epitopes belonging to the same family exhibits considerable variability. For example, Gly m4, which is also homologous to the Bet v 1 allergen in soy, is minimally affected by processing and tends to maintain its allergenicity in many highly processed soy foods. The environment and the components surrounding the allergen molecule also play a role in determining the effects of external stress on changes in protein conformational structure. The application of heat treatment resulted in a reduction in IgE reactivity of the Ara h 1 allergen in peanut, as evidenced by SDS-PAGE analysis. A comparable outcome was observed for the Ara h 2 and Ara h 3 allergens in peanut. Furthermore, a heat-resistant protomyosin of oyster origin with a molecular weight of 37 kDa was identified as a major allergen. Additionally, cooked oyster proteins show reduced IgE binding versus raw, suggesting heat-mediated allergenicity reduction [20]. Despite extensive study, boiled mussel allergenicity persists due to exceptional thermostability, lacking clinical relevance.

2. Dry Heat Processing

The application of dry heat to food products results in minimal interaction with water molecules throughout the process. The outcome of this heat treatment may be the occurrence of either a Maillard reaction or an enzymatic browning reaction. Maillard reactions entail the interaction of free amino acids present in proteins with reducing sugars (acetone and ketone), resulting in the formation of polymers that can influence the gastric digestibility of allergenic and sensitizing compounds or antigenic determinants. The IgE-binding capacity of the allergens Ara h 1 and Ara h 2 was increased about 90-fold by roasting on making peanuts undergo a Maillard reaction compared to raw peanut extracts. Consequently, the Maillard reaction of Ara h 1 and Ara h 2 resulted in a notable increase in their allergenicity [29]. However, the Maillard reaction of Pru av. 1, the primary allergen in cherries, demonstrated a reduction in their allergenicity.

3. Microwave Heating

Microwaves are electromagnetic waves with frequencies between 300 MHz and 300 GHz. These waves are employed in numerous fields, including biochemistry, medicine, and other scientific disciplines. In the food industry, microwaves are used for defrosting, pasteurizing, drying, and pre-cooking of meat frozen foods. The use of microwaves for food preparation offers numerous advantages over other heating methods. These include high heating efficiency, rapid start-up times, ease of commercial scale-up, and enhanced nutritional and sensory qualities of food. The two primary mechanisms underlying microwave heating in food are dipole rotation and ionic conduction. The presence of polar molecules is a crucial factor in the occurrence of dipole rotation. The most prevalent polar molecule in food is the water molecule, which is randomly distributed throughout the food. However, the application of microwave electric fields forces the molecules to align themselves in accordance with the direction of the electric field. The magnetic field under a microwave oven alternates at a very high frequency, and the polar molecules position themselves behind the field. The rapidly moving or rotating polar molecules interact with other molecules in the food to create friction, which results in a heating effect. Ion polarization occurs when there is a high concentration of ions present in the foodstuff. The electric field causes the ions in the food to collide with one another, whereby the kinetic energy dissipated during the collision is transformed into thermal energy. It has been measured that the high-intensity heat generated during microwave treatment can raise the temperature of the food by about 10 °C/s.

Current research on microwave heating's effects on allergens remains limited primarily to foods like fruits and soybeans. For example, an SPT-evaluated study showed that microwave treatment of kiwifruit at 40–90 °C progressively reduced allergenicity as temperature increased [30]. Following the application of microwave energy to soybeans for a period of 25 min, an allergic reaction to the processed soybeans was evidenced by the enzyme allergy susceptibility absorption test (EAST) in 9 of the 15 patients [31].

11.4.2 Biochemical Methods

Diverse nonthermal techniques—such as glycation, acid–base treatments, enzymolysis, fermentation, and other biochemical methods—are utilized in food processing. With the increasing trend of demand for commercialization of these technologies, it has become important to study the effects of these technologies on various components of food, especially on allergens. Though research remains largely in early stages, these technologies have garnered significant scholarly attention.

1. Glycosylation

Food allergens are associated with a limited number of amino acid residues, typically ranging from a few to a few dozen, within the antigenic determinant cluster of the allergen. Consequently, when these residues are masked, degraded, or removed, IgE antibodies fail to recognize allergenic epitopes—enabling production of hypoallergenic foods. A significant proportion of allergens are glycoproteins with a molecular weight of 10–80 kDa and an acidic isoelectric point. Carbohydrate moieties critically influence antigenicity, as demonstrated in multiple studies. Thus, modulating glycoprotein glycosylation represents a key strategy for reducing allergenicity. The Maillard reaction provides a primary nonenzymatic pathway for protein glycation in foods. This widespread nonenzymatic browning reaction involves carbonyl groups from reducing sugars and amino groups from proteins.

In 1912, French chemist Lewis Camilla Mallard discovered and named the Maillard reaction, a complex process accompanied by a color change [32]. The reaction results in the formation of a number of intermediates with different odors, including reduced ketones, aldehydes, and heterocyclic compounds. These compounds contribute desirable flavors and colors to foods. The Maillard reaction is operationally simple, profoundly influences food flavor and color, and is widely applied industrially. Sugar selection critically influences glycation outcomes. Commonly used sugars include glucose, maltose, lactose, and chitosan. Oligosaccharides are straight or branched-chain polysaccharides formed indirectly by 2–10 monosaccharides through glycosidic bonds. Due to their high solubility in water, oligosaccharides are also commonly used for glycosylation, such as maltose, lactose, and alginate, and are widely distributed in food and vegetable crops. Additionally, there are functional oligosaccharides, including oligofructose, oligoxylose, oligosaccharides, and cyclic oligosaccharides. Oligosaccharides alter the properties of proteins not only through glycosylation but also through direct interactions.

2. Enzymatic Processing

   Protein hydrolysis (enzymatic hydrolysis) cleaves peptide bonds within proteins' primary structures, yielding soluble peptides or amino acids. This process typically alters protein functionality, notably affecting solubility, foaming, emulsification, and hydration properties. Consequently, protein hydrolysis also results in the destruction of protein structure, thereby altering their functional properties. Furthermore, it can effectively alter the linear and conformational epitope structure of food proteins. The extent of enzymatic processing is primarily contingent upon the amino acid sequence, the secondary structure, and the structural modifications that ensue following the action of specific enzymes. The in vitro hydrolysis of the peanut allergen Ara h 2 protein resulted in a significant alteration of the secondary structure of the molecule. Yet these structural changes did not reduce sensitization because hydrolysis preserved linear epitopes. Contrasting evidence exists, as when oyster steaming modified peptide digestion profiles. Despite this, heat-stable allergen Cra g 1 retained intestinal-phase residual fragments with potential sensitizing epitopes. Two regions of Cra g 1 (residues 224–228 and 245–248) are the ones that are more tolerant in the gastrointestinal tract, and thus it is also possible that some sensitizing activity is retained.

3. Fermentation

   The process of fermentation can alter the composition of various components in food. Microorganisms, through their secretion of enzymes, can decompose macromolecular substances, such as proteins, into soluble low-molecular compounds, including small peptides and amino acids.

   Accordingly, the structure and properties of the allergens in the food are altered, and the macromolecular proteins that elicit allergic reactions in the body are inevitably affected, thereby eliminating or reducing the allergenicity. While primarily applicable to fermented foods, microbial fermentation enhances protein digestibility and contributes significantly to flavor development. This allergen-modifying effect is best documented in peanuts, soybeans, and dairy products. Studies confirm fermentation reduces allergenicity in peanut products, potentially enhancing safety. The method demonstrated a 30% reduction in the allergenicity of peanut allergens Ara h 1 and Ara h 2 with no significant impact on product quality. The consumption of fermented foods, particularly dairy products, has been demonstrated to alleviate the symptoms of certain genetic allergies and limit the development of specific diseases. Consequently, the incorporation of probiotics in milk and the creation of novel fermented products represent effective strategies for the management of allergies. Additionally, microbial fermentation has been shown to desensitize shellfish allergenic proteins and reduce the risk of sensitization.

11.4.3 Emerging Processing Methods

Most emerging food processing techniques developed in recent years are nonthermal, defined as methods that do not employ heating unless the food itself generates heat and the processing temperature is maintained below the lethal threshold. A variety of nonthermal processing techniques are employed in the food industry, including high hydrostatic pressure processing, gamma radiation (γ-ray radiation), pulsed electric field processing, and high-intensity ultrasonic processing.

1. Ultrasonic Treatment

   Ultrasonic processing utilizes mechanical waves at 20–100 kHz. The application of ultrasound results in the generation of bubbles and turbulence within the food system due to the compression and thinning effects. These bubbles subsequently collapse when they reach a critical size. Upon the collapse of the bubbles, the local temperature and pressure can reach 5000 K and 1000 atmospheres, respectively. These extreme parameters give rise to conformational changes in the protein allergenic structure. Furthermore, the high shear stresses and velocity gradients generated by micro-fluidization can also affect the composition of the food itself.

   Furthermore, the modification of proteins may be attributed to the formation of free radicals by water. Currently, there is a paucity of research examining the effects of ultrasound therapy on allergens.

   Dong et al. demonstrated high-intensity ultrasound (0–20 min, 25 °C) alters shrimp protein structure and allergenicity [33]. The results demonstrated that the allergenicity of the samples decreased with an increase in ultrasound time. The greatest reduction in allergenicity was observed at 20 min, with a 76% decrease in promyosin.

2. Irradiation Treatment

   Food irradiation technology is defined as the process of treating packaged or bulk food at a controlled dose level using gamma rays generated by ionizing radiation sources, such as Co 60 or Cs137, X-rays produced by mechanical radiation sources, or electron beams for a specified duration. At present, irradiation is employed primarily for the processing of a range of food products, including dehydrated vegetables, root vegetables, garlic, mushrooms, cereals, fruits, meat, seafood, honey, and other food items. The impact of irradiation on proteins is a complex phenomenon, with a multitude of intricate molecular mechanisms at play. The fundamental principle underlying this impact is the alteration of the high-level structure of protein molecules and the aggregation mode between protein components. This process primarily involves the induction of deamidation, decarboxylation, amino acid oxidation, the breakage or reconstruction of two sulfur bonds, and the degradation or cross-linking of peptide chains within protein molecules. Experiments have shown that small doses less than 1 kGy have little effect on the sensitizer. When the irradiation dose was greater than 1 kGy, the protein content in solution was generally reduced, except for relative molecular masses greater than 96.9 kDa. The research and application of irradiation in the removal or reduction of allergens remains in its developmental phase, and further study is required of the processes and desensitization mechanisms associated with it. Optimizing allergen inactivation while preserving food integrity warrants rigorous exploration. In addition, the complexity of the effect of strong irradiation on the activity of allergic reactions and the possibility of dose residuals from irradiation intensity are many unresolved issues that need to be further investigated.

3. Pulsed Ultraviolet (UV) Treatment

Mounting concerns about chemical preservative overuse in foods have spurred the development of alternative preservation technologies. UV radiation has been employed extensively for the purposes of water and air sanitization, as well as for the sterilization of food surfaces. Recently, it has emerged as a promising alternative to thermal and chemical treatments for shelf-life extension. The wavelength range of UV light is 100–400 nm. The effects of UV light on complex food matrices, which are composed of different ingredients, have been extensively studied as the demand for UV light in various treatments in the food industry continues to grow. Furthermore, the potential use of UV radiation as an alternative desensitization method to mitigate allergens in foods has been investigated.

11.4.4 Other Methods

Beyond glycosylation, alkaline treatments effectively modify protein allergenicity. Brenna observed that immersion in sodium hydroxide at 60 °C resulted in a reduction in the allergenic activity of peach pulp and juice [34]. Similarly, NaOH treatment diminished allergenicity in egg proteins ovalbumin and ovomucoid. As most allergens are acid-stable acidic proteins, alkaline conditions readily disrupt their structure and allergenic potential. Nevertheless, acid hydrolysis represents a chemical method for reducing the allergenicity of proteins such as wheat flour. The application of acid treatment can facilitate the alteration of the allergenic structure in wheat, thereby producing a hypoallergenic product. Treatment of gluten proteins with lactic and hydrochloric acids changed the function of glutamate residue in gluten proteins when 30% of the amide was removed, and gluten proteins showed a significant reduction in their ability to bind IgE when 50% of the amide was removed.

11.5 Summary

Rising global shellfish consumption correlates with increased allergy prevalence. Shellfish represents a significant cause of food allergies in adults and is a common trigger for such allergies. Major triggers include crustaceans (shrimp, crab, lobster) and mollusks (clams, oysters, mussels). Mollusks are frequently identified as common allergens on an international scale. Protomyosin has been identified as a primary allergen in shellfish, while arginine kinase has also been shown to be a sensitizer in some significant allergic reactions. Further research is required to enhance clinical sensitivity and species specificity for the identification of allergens, which could facilitate the definitive diagnosis of allergy. The primary method of managing shellfish allergies remains the avoidance of ingestion. Immunocompromised individuals should consume only cooked shellfish to mitigate infection risks from raw seafood pathogens. Further study of the molecular structure of protomyosin is essential for food processing to control or reduce shellfish allergenic proteins. Continued progress in the characterization of shellfish allergens will not only enhance our comprehension of the physiological basis of shellfish allergens but will also establish a foundation for the identification of food allergies and the advancement of food safety.

References

1. Renz H, Allen KJ, Sicherer SH, Sampson HA, Lack G, Beyer K, Oettgen HC. Food allergy. Nat Rev Dis Prim. 2018;4(1):1–20.
2. Pedrosa M, Boyano-Martínez T, García-Ara C, Quirce S. Shellfish allergy: a comprehensive review. Clin Rev Allergy Immunol. 2014;49(2):203–16.
3. Cheng C, Wu H, Wu C, Jan T. Pacific oyster-derived polysaccharides attenuate allergen-induced intestinal inflammation in a murine model of food allergy. J Food Drug Anal. 2016;24(1):121–8.
4. Rolland J, Varese N, Abramovitch J, Anania J, Nugraha R, Kamath S, Hazard A, Lopata A, O'Hehir R. Effect of heat processing on IgE reactivity and cross-reactivity of tropomyosin and other allergens of Asia-pacific Mollusc species: identification of novel Sydney rock oyster tropomyosin Sac g 1. Mol Nutr Food Res. 2018;62(14):1800148.
5. Liu M, Liu G, Yang Y, Mei X, Yang H, Li Y, Cao M, Liu G. Thermal processing influences the digestibility and immunoreactivity of muscle proteins of *Scylla paramamosain*. LWT-Food Sci Technol. 2018;98:559–67.
6. Taylor S. Molluscan shellfish allergy. Adv Food Nutr Res. 2008;54:139–77.
7. Zheng L, Lin H, Pawar R, Li Z, Li M. Mapping IgE binding epitopes of major shrimp allergen with immunoinformatics tools. Food Chem Toxicol. 2011;49(11):2954–60.
8. Zhang J, Liu W, Zhang R, Zhao X, Fang L, Qin X, Gu R, Lu J, Li G. Hypoallergenic mutants of the major oyster allergen Cra g 1 alleviate oyster tropomyosin allergenic potency. Int J Biol Macromol. 2020;164:1973–83.
9. Fang L, Li G, Gu R, Cai M, Lu J. Influence of thermal treatment on the characteristics of major oyster allergen Cra g 1 (tropomyosin). J Sci Food Agric. 2018;98(14):5322–8.
10. Moonesinghe H, Mackenzie H, Venter C, Kilburn S, Turner P, Weir K, Dean T. Prevalence of fish and shellfish allergy a systematic review. Ann Allerg Asthma Immunol. 2016;117(3):264.

11. Khora S. Seafood-associated shellfish allergy: a comprehensive review. Immunol Investig. 2016;45(6):504–30.
12. Lopata A, O'hehir R, Lehrer S, Allergy E. Shellfish allergy. Clin Exp Allergy. 2010;40(6):850–8.
13. Ishikawa M, Shimakura K, Nagashima Y, Shiomi K. Isolation and properties of allergenic proteins in the oyster Crassostrea gigas. Fish Sci. 1997;63(4):610–4.
14. Fu L, Song J, Wang C, Fu S, Wang Y. Potentially alleviates shrimp tropomyosin-induced allergy by Tolerogenic dendritic cell-dependent induction of regulatory T cells and alterations in gut microbiota. Front Immunol. 2017;8:1536.
15. Zhang Y, Chen H, Maleki S, Cao M, Zhang L, Su W, Liu G. Purification, characterization, and analysis of the allergenic properties of myosin light chain in *Procambarus clarkii*. J Agric Food Chem. 2015;63(27):6271–82.
16. Yang Y, Hu M, Jin T, Zhang Y, Liu G, Li Y, Zhang M, Cao M, Su W, Liu G. A comprehensive analysis of the allergenicity and IgE epitopes of myosinogen allergens in. Clin Exp Allergy. 2019;49(1):108–19.
17. Yang Y, Liu G, Yang H, Hu M, Cao M, Su W, Jin T, Liu G. Crystal structure determination of arginine kinase, an allergen that may cause cross-reactivity among invertebrates. Food Chem. 2019;271:597–605.
18. Yuan F, Lv L, Li Z, Mi N, Chen H, Lin H. Effect of transglutaminase-catalyzed glycosylation on the allergenicity and conformational structure of shrimp tropomyosin. Food Chem. 2017;219:215–22.
19. Fu L, Wang J, Ni S, Wang C, Wang Y. Identification of allergenic epitopes and critical amino acids of major allergens in Chinese shrimp by Immunoinformatics coupled with competitive-binding strategy. J Agric Food Chem. 2018;66(11):2944–53.
20. Suh S, Kim M, Kim H, Kim H, Kim H. A multiplex PCR assay combined with capillary electrophoresis for the simultaneous detection of tropomyosin allergens from oyster, mussel, abalone, and clam mollusk species. Food Chem. 2020;317:126451.
21. Korte R, Monneuse J, Gemrot E, Metton I, Humpf H, Brockmeyer J. New high-performance liquid chromatography coupled mass spectrometry method for the detection of lobster and shrimp allergens in food samples *via* multiple reaction monitoring and multiple reaction monitoring cubed. J Agric Food Chem. 2016;64(31):6219–27.
22. Taguchi H, Watanabe S, Temmei Y, Hirao T, Akiyama H, Sakai S, Adachi R, Sakata K, Urisu A, Teshima R. Differential detection of shrimp and crab for food labeling using polymerase chain reaction. J Agric Food Chem. 2011;59(8):3510–9.
23. Eischeid A. Development and evaluation of a real-time PCR assay for detection of lobster, a crustacean shellfish allergen. Food Control. 2016;59:393–9.
24. Vanga S, Singh A, Raghavan V. Review of conventional and novel food processing methods on food allergens. Crit Rev Food Sci Nutr. 2017;57(10):2077–94.
25. Fu L, Ni S, Wang C, Wang Y. Transglutaminase-catalysed cross-linking eliminates tropomyosin allergenicity by altering protein structure. Food Agric Immunol. 2019;30(1):296–308.
26. Gruber P, Vieths S, Wangorsch A, Nerkamp J, Hofmann T. Maillard reaction and enzymatic browning affect the allergenicity of Pru av 1, the major allergen from cherry (*Prunus avium*). J Agric Food Chem. 2004;52(12):4002–7.
27. Szamos J, Takács K, Szabó E, Kovács E, Gelencsér É. Purification of natural Mal d 1 and Mal d 2 allergens and monitoring of their expression levels during ripening in Golden Delicious apple. Food Res Int. 2011;44(9):2674–8.
28. Rib-Schmidt C, Riedl P, Meisinger V, Schwaben L, Schulenborg T, Reuter A, Schiller D, Seutter von Loetzen C, Rösch P. pH and heat resistance of the major celery allergen Api g 1. Mol Nutr Food Res. 2018;62(15):e1700886.
29. Maleki S, Chung S, Champagne E, Raufman J, Immunology C. The effects of roasting on the allergenic properties of peanut proteins. J Allergy Clin Immunol. 2000;106(4):763–8.
30. Wang J, Zhang L, Shi J, Vanga S, Raghavan V. Effect of microwave processing on the nutritional properties and allergenic potential of kiwifruit. Food Chem. 2023;401:134189.

31. Besler M, Steinhart H, Paschke A. Stability of food allergens and allergenicity of processed foods. J Chromatogr B. 2001;756(1–2):207–28.
32. Han X, Yang H, Rao S, Liu G, Hu M, Zeng B, Cao M, Liu G. The Maillard reaction reduced the sensitization of tropomyosin and arginine kinase from, simultaneously. J Agric Food Chem. 2018;66(11):2934–43.
33. Dong X, Wang J, Raghavan V. Effects of high-intensity ultrasound processing on the physiochemical and allergenic properties of shrimp. Innovative Food Sci Emerg Technol. 2020;65:102441.
34. Brenna O, Pompei C, Ortolani C, Pravettoni V, Pastorello EA, Farioli L. Technological processes to decrease the allergenicity of peach juice and nectar. J Agric Food Chem. 2000;48(2):493–7.

MIX
Papier aus verantwortungsvollen Quellen
Paper from responsible sources
FSC® C105338

If you have any concerns about our products,
you can contact us on
ProductSafety@springernature.com

In case Publisher is established outside the EU,
the EU authorized representative is:
Springer Nature Customer Service Center GmbH
Europaplatz 3, 69115 Heidelberg, Germany

Printed by Libri Plureos GmbH
in Hamburg, Germany